Prevention of endocarditis

2008

Update from *Therapeutic Guidelines: Antibiotic* version 13, and *Therapeutic Guidelines: Oral and Dental* version 1.

Copyright © 2008 Therapeutic Guidelines Limited

All rights reserved. Apart from any fair dealing for the purpose of private study, criticism, or review as permitted under the *Copyright Act 1968*, no part of this publication may be reproduced, stored in a retrieval system, scanned or transmitted in any form without the permission of the copyright owner.

Suggested citation:

Infective Endocarditis Prophylaxis Expert Group. Prevention of endocarditis. 2008 update from Therapeutic guidelines: antibiotic version 13, and Therapeutic guidelines: oral and dental version 1. Melbourne: Therapeutic Guidelines Limited; 2008.

Revised 2008

Publisher and distributor:
Therapeutic Guidelines Limited
Ground Floor, 23–47 Villiers Street
North Melbourne, Victoria 3051
Australia

Telephone: (03) 9329 1566
Facsimile: (03) 9326 5632
Freecall: 1800 061 260
Email: sales@tg.com.au
Website: http://www.tg.com.au

Printing: McPherson's Printing Group

Prevention of endocarditis

GENERAL CONSIDERATIONS

Infective endocarditis is an uncommon illness with a high morbidity and mortality. For many years antibiotic prophylaxis has been given routinely before dental and other procedures to patients with cardiac conditions that carry a high lifetime risk of infective endocarditis. However, the evidence suggests that endocarditis after dental or other procedures is infrequent and hence prophylaxis prevents very few cases. Infective endocarditis is more likely to result from bacteraemias associated with daily activities and so the maintenance of good oral health and hygiene is more important than peri-procedural antibiotics.

No randomised controlled trial has been performed to decide the role of antibiotic prophylaxis and there are no human studies showing that it can prevent endocarditis. Guidelines produced in different parts of the world rely on expert consensus and consequently can differ in their recommendations. These Australian guidelines follow the lead of the American Heart Association*, continuing a trend to reduce the categories of patients for whom prophylaxis is recommended while still specifying procedures for which prophylaxis is required.

Antibiotic prophylaxis is now recommended only for patients with cardiac conditions associated with the highest risk of *adverse outcomes* from endocarditis (see Box 1, p.2) if undergoing a specified dental (see Table 1, p.4) or other procedure (see Table 2, p.6; Table 3, p.8; Table 4, p.9). This list of cardiac conditions is short and all of these patients have had significant cardiovascular diseases or interventions. Prophylaxis is no longer recommended for patients with other forms of valvular or structural heart disease, including mitral valve prolapse.

---

* Wilson W, Taubert KA, Gewitz M, Lockhart PB, Baddour LM, Levison M, et al. Prevention of infective endocarditis: guidelines from the American Heart Association: a guideline from the American Heart Association Rheumatic Fever, Endocarditis, and Kawasaki Disease Committee, Council on Cardiovascular Disease in the Young, and the Council on Clinical Cardiology, Council on Cardiovascular Surgery and Anesthesia, and the Quality of Care and Outcomes Research Interdisciplinary Working Group. Circulation 2007;116(15):1736-54.

> **Box 1. Cardiac conditions associated with the highest risk of adverse outcomes from endocarditis**
>
> **Antibiotic prophylaxis is recommended in patients with the following cardiac conditions if undergoing a specified dental (see Table 1, p.4) or other procedure (see Table 2, p.6; Table 3, p.8; Table 4, p.9):**
>
> - prosthetic cardiac valve or prosthetic material used for cardiac valve repair
> - previous infective endocarditis
> - congenital heart disease *but* only if it involves:
>   - unrepaired cyanotic defects, including palliative shunts and conduits
>   - completely repaired defects with prosthetic material or devices, whether placed by surgery or catheter intervention, during the first 6 months after the procedure (after which the prosthetic material is likely to have been endothelialised)
>   - repaired defects with residual defects at or adjacent to the site of a prosthetic patch or device (which inhibit endothelialisation)
> - cardiac transplantation with the subsequent development of cardiac valvulopathy
> - rheumatic heart disease in Indigenous Australians only

It is recognised that the change in recommendations, while justified and in progression from past guidelines, may appear to be controversial. In certain individual circumstances, medical and dental practitioners may consider giving antibiotics to patients not covered by these guidelines. These include patients who have received prophylactic antibiotics over their lifetime and are unwilling to change this practice.

In addition, Indigenous Australian patients with rheumatic heart disease may be a special population at high risk for infective endocarditis or for adverse outcomes from endocarditis. Accordingly, this group has also been included in the list of patients with cardiac conditions requiring prophylaxis (see Box 1, above).

All patients with cardiac abnormalities should be reminded to practise good oral hygiene and have regular dental evaluation. In particular, dental examination is recommended twice yearly for patients with cardiac conditions involving the endocardium, especially those listed in Box 1. Doctors should be alert to investigate an unexplained fever which could be a sign of endocarditis, and take blood cultures before any oral or intravenous antibiotics are administered.

PROCEDURES AND ANTIBIOTIC RECOMMENDATIONS

Dental procedures

Bacteraemia associated with dental procedures predominantly involves viridans group streptococci, organisms known to cause infective endocarditis. Traditionally, the presence of 'significant bleeding' associated with a dental procedure has been taken as an indication of bacteraemia and hence need for prophylaxis; however, bleeding has been shown to be a poor indicator of bacteraemia from dental procedures.

The key parameters of a bacteraemia are its incidence, magnitude and duration. The magnitude and duration of the bacteraemia are dependent on the state of periodontal health, the vigour of the dentogingival or apical manipulation and the duration of the procedure. Some procedures may or may not require prophylaxis depending on these factors.

Prophylaxis is always required for those procedures with a high incidence of bacteraemia (may occur in 70% or more patients). Dental procedures with a moderate incidence of bacteraemia (may occur in 30% or more patients) should be considered for prophylaxis depending on the circumstances of the procedure and the periodontal condition (see Table 1, p.4). Thus, for example, periodontal probing on a single healthy tooth would not justify antibiotic prophylaxis whereas full-mouth periodontal probing on a patient with periodontitis would.

Prophylaxis is not recommended for procedures with a low incidence of bacteraemia.

Patient-performed oral hygiene activities, such as toothbrushing, flossing or use of oral irrigators, can produce similar incidences of bacteraemia as that caused by most dental procedures (excluding extractions and subgingival scaling/root planing). As these activities are performed more frequently, they have the potential to produce regular episodes of bacteraemia, particularly in patients with gingival inflammation. It is considered that the cumulative effect of repeated episodes of bacteraemia caused by oral hygiene activities is very likely to be a more important risk factor for infective endocarditis than isolated episodes of bacteraemia occurring during dental visits, especially in patients with poor oral health and hygiene.

Table 1. Dental procedures and their requirement for endocarditis prophylaxis in patients with cardiac conditions listed in Box 1

Prophylaxis always required	Prophylaxis required in some circumstances	Prophylaxis not required
<ul><li>extraction</li><li>periodontal procedures including surgery, subgingival scaling and root planing</li><li>replanting avulsed teeth</li><li>other surgical procedures (eg implant placement, apicoectomy)</li></ul>	*Consider prophylaxis for the following procedures if multiple procedures are being conducted, the procedure is prolonged or periodontal disease is present:* <ul><li>full periodontal probing for patients with periodontitis</li><li>intraligamentary and intraosseous local anaesthetic injection</li><li>supragingival calculus removal/cleaning</li><li>rubber dam placement with clamps (where risk of damaging gingiva)</li><li>restorative matrix band/strip placement</li><li>endodontics beyond the apical foramen</li><li>placement of orthodontic bands</li><li>placement of interdental wedges</li><li>subgingival placement of retraction cords, antibiotic fibres or antibiotic strips</li></ul>	<ul><li>oral examination</li><li>infiltration and block local anaesthetic injection</li><li>restorative dentistry</li><li>supragingival rubber dam clamping and placement of rubber dam</li><li>intracanal endodontic procedures</li><li>removal of sutures</li><li>impressions and construction of dentures</li><li>orthodontic bracket placement and adjustment of fixed appliances</li><li>application of gels</li><li>intraoral radiographs</li><li>supragingival plaque removal</li></ul>

If after careful evaluation of both the cardiac condition (see Box 1, p.2) and the dental procedure (see Table 1, above), antibiotic prophylaxis is considered necessary, a single dose of antibiotic should be given before the procedure; there is no proven value to giving a follow-up dose 6 hours later.

If a patient is having more than one procedure requiring antibiotic prophylaxis, dentists should carefully consider their treatment plan and modify it as necessary so that all of the procedures can be completed in a single or at most two sittings, thus avoiding the need for multiple antibiotic doses.

For standard prophylaxis, use:

> *amoxycillin 2 g (child: 50 mg/kg up to 2 g) orally, 1 hour before the procedure*
> *or amoxy/ampicillin 2 g (child: 50 mg/kg up to 2 g) IV, just before the procedure*
> *or amoxy/ampicillin 2 g (child: 50 mg/kg up to 2 g) IM, 30 minutes before the procedure.*

Patients hypersensitive to penicillin, and those on long-term penicillin therapy or who have taken penicillin or a related beta-lactam antibiotic more than once in the previous month, can use:

1. *clindamycin 600 mg (child: 15 mg/kg up to 600 mg) orally, 1 hour before the procedure*
   or clindamycin 600 mg (child: 15 mg/kg up to 600 mg) IV over at least 20 minutes, just before the procedure

   OR

1. *lincomycin 600 mg (child: 15 mg/kg up to 600 mg) IV over at least 1 hour, just before the procedure*

   OR

2. *vancomycin 25 mg/kg up to 1.5 g (child less than 12 years: 30 mg/kg up to 1.5 g) IV by slow infusion (over at least 60 minutes; rate not exceeding 10 mg/min), ending the infusion just before the procedure*

   OR

3. *teicoplanin 400 mg (child: 10 mg/kg up to 400 mg) IV, just before the procedure*
   or teicoplanin 400 mg (child: 10 mg/kg up to 400 mg) IM, 30 minutes before the procedure.

There is no oral liquid formulation of clindamycin in Australia. An alternative for patients who are hypersensitive to penicillin (excluding immediate hypersensitivity), is:

cephalexin 2 g (child: 50 mg/kg up to 2 g) orally, 1 hour before the procedure.

Cephalexin is not suitable for those who have been on long-term penicillin or have taken a related beta-lactam antibiotic more than once in the previous month.

Respiratory tract procedures

Bacteraemia associated with respiratory procedures predominantly involves viridans group streptococci, organisms known to cause infective endocarditis. Prophylaxis is only recommended for those procedures which have an increased risk of bacteraemia (see Table 2, below).

Table 2. Respiratory tract procedures and their requirement for endocarditis prophylaxis in patients with cardiac conditions listed in Box 1

Prophylaxis always required (high risk of bacteraemia)	Prophylaxis not required (low risk of bacteraemia)
Any invasive procedure involving incision or biopsy of respiratory mucosa—for example: • tonsillectomy/adenoidectomy • rigid or flexible bronchoscopy *with* incision or biopsy • surgery involving bronchial, sinus, nasal or middle ear mucosa, including tympanostomy tube insertion	*These are examples of situations where prophylaxis of infective endocarditis would not be required:* • rigid or flexible bronchoscopy *without* incision or biopsy • endotracheal intubation

If after careful evaluation of both the cardiac condition (see Box 1, p.2) and the respiratory tract procedure (see Table 2, above), antibiotic prophylaxis is considered necessary, a single dose of antibiotic should be given before the procedure; there is no proven value to giving a follow-up dose 6 hours later. For standard prophylaxis, antibiotic choice is the same as for dental procedures (see antibiotic recommendations under Dental procedures, p.5).

Genitourinary and gastrointestinal tract procedures

Bacteraemia associated with genitourinary and gastrointestinal procedures predominantly involves enteroccoci, organisms known to cause infective endocarditis.

In patients with cardiac conditions listed in Box 1, prophylaxis is generally only recommended for genitourinary and gastrointestinal procedures which, because of their increased risk of bacteraemia, also have an indication for antibiotic prophylaxis for surgical reasons (eg to prevent wound infection or sepsis) (see Table 3, p.8). The recommended antibiotic for infective endocarditis prophylaxis should be given *in addition to* the antibiotic required for surgical prophylaxis (see Prophylaxis: surgical in *Therapeutic Guidelines: Antibiotic* version 13).

Infective endocarditis prophylaxis is also recommended for lithotripsy and vaginal delivery with prolonged labour in patients with cardiac conditions listed in Box 1. These procedures similarly have an increased risk of bacteraemia.

Also, for patients with an established genitourinary or intra-abdominal infection undergoing a related procedure and who have a cardiac condition listed in Box 1, *additional* infective endocarditis prophylaxis is required with an antibiotic active against enterococci (see antibiotic recommendations below) unless such an antibiotic is already part of the treatment regimen.

If after careful consideration of both the cardiac condition (see Box 1, p.2) and the genitourinary or gastrointestinal procedure (see Table 3, p.8), antibiotic prophylaxis is considered necessary, use:

amoxy/ampicillin 2 g (child: 50 mg/kg up to 2 g) IV, just before the procedure
or amoxy/ampicillin 2 g (child: 50 mg/kg up to 2 g) IM, 30 minutes before the procedure.

For patients with immediate penicillin hypersensitivity, use:

1. *vancomycin 25 mg/kg up to 1.5 g (child less than 12 years: 30 mg/kg up to 1.5 g) IV by slow infusion (over at least 60 minutes; rate not exceeding 10 mg/min), ending the infusion just before the procedure*

   OR

2. *teicoplanin 400 mg (child: 10 mg/kg up to 400 mg) IV, just before the procedure.*

Table 3. Genitourinary and gastrointestinal tract procedures and their requirement for endocarditis prophylaxis in patients with cardiac conditions listed in Box 1

Prophylaxis always required (high risk of bacteraemia)	Prophylaxis not required (low risk of bacteraemia)

• any procedure where antibiotic prophylaxis is indicated for surgical reasons (see Prophylaxis: surgical in *Therapeutic Guidelines: Antibiotic* version 13)
• lithotripsy
• vaginal delivery with prolonged labour
• any genitourinary procedure in the presence of a genitourinary infection unless already treating enterococci (for *elective* cystoscopy or urinary tract manipulations, obtain a urine culture and treat any significant bacteriuria beforehand)
• any gastrointestinal procedure in the presence of an intra-abdominal infection unless already treating enteroccoci
	• procedures not requiring surgical prophylaxis and in the absence of related infection. *Examples include:*
	  – urethral catheterisation, uterine dilatation and curettage, sterilisation procedures, insertion or removal of intrauterine contraceptive device
	  – vaginal delivery
	  – transoesophageal echocardiography
	  – endoscopy +/– biopsy, including colonoscopy
	  – percutaneous endoscopic gastrostomy

Other procedures

For patients who have a cardiac condition associated with a high risk of adverse outcomes from infective endocarditis (see Box 1, p.2) and who are undergoing a procedure listed in Table 4, it is particularly important that antibiotic treatment should be given as recommended for the specific procedure (see cross-references in Table 4 below).

Table 4. Other procedures which require antibiotic treatment in patients with cardiac conditions listed in Box 1*

- incision and drainage of local abscess:
  - brain (see Brain abscess or subdural empyema, p.65)
  - boils and carbuncles (see Boils and carbuncles, p.271)
  - dacryocystitis (see Dacryocystitis, p.71)
  - epidural (see Epidural abscess, p.66)
  - lung (see Lung abscess, p.226)
  - orbital (see Orbital [postseptal] cellulitis, p.71)
  - perirectal (see Perirectal abscess, p.90)
  - pyogenic liver (see Pyogenic liver abscess, p.144)
  - tooth (see Acute odontogenic infections, p.167)
- surgical procedures through infected skin (see Cellulitis, p.274)

* The page numbers for cross-references refer to the relevant topics in *Therapeutic Guidelines: Antibiotic* version 13

Infective Endocarditis Prophylaxis Expert Group

Professor Robert Moulds (chairman)
Professor of Medicine, Fiji School of Medicine
Suva, Fiji

Professor Bart Currie
Head, Infectious Diseases Program, Menzies School of Health Research and Royal Darwin Hospital
Casuarina, Northern Territory

Associate Professor Christopher Daly
Associate Professor of Periodontology, Faculty of Dentistry, The University of Sydney
Sydney, New South Wales

Professor Alastair Goss
Professor of Oral and Maxillofacial Surgery,
The University of Adelaide
Director of Oral and Maxillofacial Surgery, Adelaide Dental Hospital and Royal Adelaide Hospital
Adelaide, South Australia

Ms Melanie Jeyasingham
Editor, Therapeutic Guidelines Limited
Melbourne, Victoria

Professor Julian Smith
Professor of Surgery, Monash University
Head, Cardiothoracic Surgery Unit, Monash Medical Centre
Clayton, Victoria

Associate Professor Neil Strathmore
Associate Professor, The University of Melbourne
Cardiologist, The Royal Melbourne Hospital
Melbourne, Victoria

Dr Alan Street
Deputy Director, Victorian Infectious Disease Service, The Royal Melbourne Hospital
Melbourne, Victoria

Members of the expert group complied with Therapeutic Guidelines Limited policy on conflict of interest. For more information see <http://www.tg.com.au/index.php?sectionid=38>.

Acknowledgments

The manuscript has been previewed by the following individuals to whom we express appreciation and thanks:

Associate Professor Roger Allan
Cardiac Services Clinical Stream Director, South Eastern Sydney Illawarra Health, New South Wales

Professor Peter Collignon
Director of Microbiology and Infectious Diseases, Canberra Hospital, Australian Capital Territory
Professor, Australian National University Medical School, Australian Capital Territory

Dr Jennifer Johns
Cardiologist, Medical Director, Specialty Services CSU, Austin Health, Victoria

Dr John Matthews
President, Australian Dental Association Inc.
General Dental Practitioner, Victoria

Associate Professor Michael McCullough
Oral Medicine, School of Dental Science,
The University of Melbourne, Victoria

Endorsements

Australasian Society for Infectious Diseases (ASID)
Australian College of Rural and Remote Medicine (ACRRM)
Australian Dental Association Inc.
Australian Society for Antimicrobials
The Cardiac Society of Australia and New Zealand (CSANZ)
Heart Foundation
National Prescribing Service Limited (NPS)
Royal Australasian College of Dental Surgeons (RACDS)
School of Dental Science, The University of Melbourne
School of Dentistry, The University of Adelaide
School of Dentistry, The University of Queensland
School of Dentistry, The University of Western Australia
The Royal Australian College of General Practitioners (RACGP)
The Society of Hospital Pharmacists of Australia (SHPA)

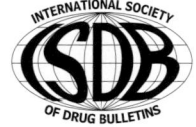

Therapeutic Guidelines Limited.

ABN 45 074 766 224

Ground Floor, 23-47 Villiers Street,
North Melbourne, Victoria 3051, Australia

FREECALL 1800 061 260
PH +61 3 9329 1566   **FAX** +61 3 9326 5632
EMAIL sales@tg.com.au   www.tg.com.au

Therapeutic Guidelines

Oral and Dental

Many thanks for your support and involvement in the 2009 AMSA Global Health Conference

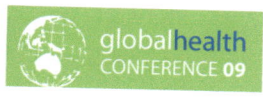

*From the GHC Committee
Brisbane, 2009*

Other guidelines
available from Therapeutic Guidelines Limited

Therapeutic Guidelines: Analgesic
Therapeutic Guidelines: Antibiotic
Therapeutic Guidelines: Cardiovascular
Therapeutic Guidelines: Dermatology
Therapeutic Guidelines: Endocrinology
Therapeutic Guidelines: Gastrointestinal
Therapeutic Guidelines: Neurology
Therapeutic Guidelines: Palliative Care
Therapeutic Guidelines: Psychotropic
Therapeutic Guidelines: Respiratory
Therapeutic Guidelines: Rheumatology
Management Guidelines: Developmental Disability
eTG complete
miniTG

Therapeutic Guidelines

Oral and Dental

2007
VERSION 1

Oral and Dental Expert Group

Therapeutic Guidelines Limited, Melbourne

with

Australian Dental Association

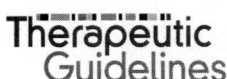 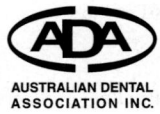

Copyright © 2007 Therapeutic Guidelines Limited

All rights reserved. Apart from any fair dealing for the purpose of private study, criticism, or review as permitted under the *Copyright Act 1968*, no part of this publication may be reproduced, stored in a retrieval system, scanned or transmitted in any form without the permission of the copyright owner.

Suggested citation:
Oral and Dental Expert Group. Therapeutic guidelines: oral and dental. Version 1. Melbourne: Therapeutic Guidelines Limited; 2007.

First published 2007
Reprinted 2008

Published by
Therapeutic Guidelines Limited
Ground Floor, 23–47 Villiers Street
North Melbourne, Victoria 3051
Australia

Telephone: (03) 9329 1566
Facsimile: (03) 9326 5632
Freecall: 1800 061 260
Email: sales@tg.com.au
Website: http://www.tg.com.au

National Library of Australia Cataloguing-in-Publication data:

Therapeutic guidelines: oral and dental
Version 1.
Includes index.

ISBN 978 0 9757393 6 5 (pbk)

ISBN 0 9757393 6 0 (pbk)

1. Dental therapeutics - Handbooks, manuals, etc.
I. Therapeutic Guidelines Limited. Oral and Dental Expert Group

617.606

Printing: McPherson's Printing Group

Contents

Tables, boxes, figures and photos vii
Oral and Dental Expert Group xi
Acknowledgments xiii
Endorsements xvi
About Therapeutic Guidelines Limited xvii
Preface xxv

Chapters
Principles of diagnosis and prescribing 1
Prescriptions and prescription-writing 5
Getting to know your drugs 13
Dental management of patients taking medications 61
Dental caries 91
Periodontal disease 97
Halitosis 103
Oral mucosal disease 107
Acute odontogenic infections 127
Antibiotic prophylaxis 135
Post-treatment pain management 145
Local anaesthesia 157
Oral sedation 161
Medical emergencies 165

Appendices
Appendix 1. Drugs and sport 191
Appendix 2. Dental procedures and drugs during pregnancy and breastfeeding 193

Abbreviations and acronyms 203

Glossary 205

Index 219

Request for comment on guidelines 235

Tables, boxes, figures and photos

Tables

Table 1.	Antimicrobial drugs used in dentistry	16
Table 2.	Adverse effects of nonsteroidal anti-inflammatory drugs	31
Table 3.	Adverse effects of opioids	35
Table 4.	Properties of topical corticosteroids used on the oral mucosa	40
Table 5.	Properties of local anaesthetic groups	46
Table 6.	Duration of action and maximum doses of local anaesthetics used in dentistry	50
Table 7.	Risk of osteonecrosis of the jaws in patients taking bisphosphonates	77
Table 8.	Drugs commonly used in psychiatric disorders	89
Table 9.	Examples of topical applications and how they may be used for caries reduction in patients at elevated risk of developing caries	95
Table 10.	Causes of mouth ulceration	114
Table 11.	Predisposing factors in oral candidosis	119
Table 12.	Oral preparations available for mucositis and xerostomia	123
Table 13.	Cardiac conditions that have a risk for infective endocarditis with dental procedures	136
Table 14.	Dental procedures and their risk of causing a bacteraemia	137
Table 15.	Need for antibiotic prophylaxis for patients with a cardiac condition undergoing a dental procedure	138
Table 16.	Advantages and disadvantages of oral sedation	161
Table 17.	Initial assessment of the severity of an acute attack of asthma	172
Table 18.	Signs of obstruction	174
Table 19.	Drug use in pregnancy and breastfeeding	197

Boxes

Box 1.	General principles of treating disease	1
Box 2.	Aspects of the examination and diagnosis that should be included in clinical records	3
Box 3.	Principles of use of antibiotics	14
Box 4.	The antibiotic creed	14
Box 5.	Risk factors for developing NSAID-associated gastrointestinal adverse reactions	32
Box 6.	Points to consider when prescribing topical corticosteroids	39
Box 7.	Procedure for patients taking warfarin who require minor oral surgery	64
Box 8.	Routine dental treatment for a patient with stable diabetes	73
Box 9.	History-taking relating to bisphosphonates	76
Box 10.	Some common causes of halitosis	104
Box 11.	Treatment options for localised acute odontogenic infections	128
Box 12.	Recommendations for dental treatment of patients with artificial joint replacement	142
Box 13.	Combining the use of ibuprofen with paracetamol+codeine for enhanced pain management in adults	152
Box 14.	How the recommendations for pain management were derived	154
Box 15.	Instructions for patients having oral sedation	163
Box 16.	Management of syncope	167
Box 17.	Management of angina	168
Box 18.	Management of suspected acute myocardial infarction	169
Box 19.	Management of cardiac arrest	170
Box 20.	Management of hyperventilation syndrome	171
Box 21.	Management of acute asthma	173
Box 22.	Management of an inhaled or swallowed object	174

Box 23.	Management of stroke	176
Box 24.	Management of seizures	177
Box 25.	Management of hypoglycaemia	178
Box 26.	Management of diabetic ketoacidosis	179
Box 27.	Management of Addisonian (adrenal) crisis	179
Box 28.	Management of urticaria	182
Box 29.	Management of anaphylactoid and anaphylactic reactions	183
Box 30.	Medical management of severe anaphylactoid and anaphylactic reactions	184

Figures

Figure 1.	Example of the format required for a legal prescription	9
Figure 2.	Schematic diagram of some odontogenic infections and the stages of dental caries (decay)	128
Figure 3.	Conceptual figure showing the relationship of dental procedure to bacteraemia and the threshold for antibiotic prophylaxis	139
Figure 4.	Schematic representation of blood levels of drugs taken alternately for the management of severe pain	152
Figure 5.	Example of instructions for a patient following surgery (using a timeline)	153
Figure 6.	Schematic representation of pain relief with different systemic medications using the 'third molar model'	154
Figure 7.	Basic life support flow chart	187

Photos

Photo 1.	Leukoplakia	108
Photo 2.	Squamous cell carcinoma	109
Photo 3.	Oral lichen planus	110
Photo 4.	Oral hairy leukoplakia	112
Photo 5.	Traumatic ulcer	113
Photo 6.	Mucous membrane pemphigoid	117

Oral and Dental Expert Group

Dr J Dowden (Chairman)
Editor-in-Chief, Australian Prescriber, Deakin, Australian Capital Territory

Professor Paul Abbott
Professor of Clinical Dentistry, Head of the School of Dentistry, Director of the Oral Health Centre of Western Australia, Deputy Dean of the Faculty of Medicine, Dentistry and Health Sciences, The University of Western Australia
Endodontist, Perth, Western Australia

Professor Alastair N Goss
Professor Oral and Maxillofacial Surgery, The University of Adelaide
Director of Oral and Maxillofacial Surgery, Adelaide Dental Hospital and Royal Adelaide Hospital, South Australia

Associate Professor Michael McCullough
Oral Medicine, School of Dental Science, The University of Melbourne, Victoria

Dr John Matthews
Vice-president, Australian Dental Association
General Practitioner, Essendon, Victoria

Dr Jill Pope
Editor, Therapeutic Guidelines Limited, Melbourne, Victoria

Associate Professor Louis Roller
Department of Pharmacy Practice, Associate Dean (Teaching), Faculty of Pharmacy, Monash University, Melbourne, Victoria

Associate Professor Neil Savage
Reader, Oral Medicine and Pathology, The University of Queensland
Consultant Oral Pathologist, Royal Brisbane and Women's Hospital, Queensland

Associate Professor Marc Tennant
Director, Centre for Rural and Remote Oral Health, The University of Western Australia

Acknowledgments

The entire manuscript has been previewed by the following individuals to whom we express appreciation and thanks:

Associate Professor Hedley Coleman
Oral Pathologist, Westmead Hospital, The University of Sydney, New South Wales

Dr Rhonda Gwyther
Dental Practitioner, Essendon, Victoria

Dr Mark Hutton
Dental Practitioner, Mount Gambier, South Australia

Professor Andrew McLachlan
Faculty of Pharmacy, The University of Sydney, and Centre for Education and Research on Ageing, Concord Hospital, New South Wales

Dr Paul Sambrook
Senior Lecturer, School of Dentistry, The University of Adelaide, South Australia

The following sections were prepared in consultation with the expert group for *Therapeutic Guidelines: Antibiotic* version 13:

Acute odontogenic infections

Antibiotic prophylaxis

Periodontal disease

The expert group thanks the following individuals for contributing to the following sections:

Local anaesthesia
Dr Shiva Subramaniam
Dental Practitioner, Centre for Rural and Remote Oral Health, The University of Western Australia

Oral sedation
Associate Professor Ray Williamson
Oral Health Centre, The University of Western Australia

Periodontal disease
Dr Rod Marshall
Senior Lecturer in Periodontology, School of Dentistry, The University of Queensland

The expert group thanks colleagues who have contributed to these guidelines either directly through draft text, advice or criticism, or indirectly through views expressed in committees and discussions. We would particularly like to thank the following:

Dr Helen Boocock
Lecturer, School of Dentistry, The University of Queensland

Dr Louise Brown
Periodontist, Melbourne, Victoria

Dr Stephen Cottrell
Periodontist, Department of Maxillofacial Surgery, The Royal Melbourne Hospital, Victoria

Associate Professor Christopher Daly
Discipline of Periodontics, Faculty of Dentistry, The University of Sydney, New South Wales

Dr John Fahey
Managing Director, Cynergex Group Pty Ltd, Sydney, New South Wales

Emeritus Professor Ken Ilett
School of Medicine and Pharmacology, The University of Western Australia, Perth, Western Australia

Ms Judith Kristensen
Senior Pharmacist, King Edward Memorial Hospital for Women, Perth, Western Australia

Dr Richard Logan
Senior Lecturer and Head of Oral Pathology, School of Dentistry, The University of Adelaide, South Australia

Dr James Lucas
Paediatric Dentist, Deputy, Director Department of Dentistry, Royal Children's Hospital, Melbourne, Victoria

Ms Jenny McDowell
Research Officer, Department of Pharmacy Practice, Victorian College of Pharmacy, Monash University, Melbourne, Victoria

Dr John McIntyre
Visiting Research Fellow, Dental School, The University of Adelaide, South Australia

Professor Stanley Malamed
Dentist Anesthesiologist, Section of Anesthesia and Medicine, University of Southern California, School of Dentistry, Los Angeles, United States of America

Mr Stephen Marty
Registrar, Pharmacy Board of Victoria

Professor Eric Reynolds
Head, School of Dental Science and CEO, Centre for Oral Health Science, The University of Melbourne, Victoria

Dr Alison Rich
Senior Lecturer in Oral Pathology, Associate Dean Undergraduate Studies, School of Dentistry, University of Otago, Dunedin, New Zealand

Dr Mark Schifter
Specialist, Oral Medicine Unit, Centre for Oral Health, Westmead, New South Wales

Dr Margaret Stacey
Lecturer, School of Dental Science, The University of Melbourne, Victoria

Dr Nandor Steidler
Oral and Maxillofacial Surgeon, Melbourne, Victoria

Dr Russell Vickers
Clinical Senior Lecturer, Faculty of Medicine, The University of Sydney, New South Wales

Professor Laurie Walsh
Head, School of Dentistry, The University of Queensland

Dr Gavin Wheaton
Paediatric Cardiologist, Adelaide Women's and Children's Hospital, South Australia

Mr David Wiesenfeld
Head of Oral and Maxillofacial Surgery Unit, The Royal Melbourne Hospital, Victoria

Endorsements

Australian College of Rural and Remote Medicine (ACRRM)
Faculty of Dentistry, The University of Sydney
National Heart Foundation of Australia
National Prescribing Service Limited (NPS)
Royal Australasian College of Dental Surgeons
School of Dental Science, The University of Melbourne
School of Dentistry, The University of Adelaide
School of Dentistry, The University of Queensland
School of Dentistry, The University of Western Australia
The Royal Australian College of General Practitioners (RACGP)
The Society of Hospital Pharmacists of Australia (SHPA)

Professor Newell W Johnson
Foundation Dean and Head of School, School of Dentistry and Oral Health, Griffith University

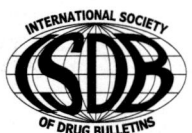

About Therapeutic Guidelines Limited

KEY INFORMATION ABOUT THESE GUIDELINES

Dosing regimens

The regimens in the text apply, when not otherwise specified, to average-sized, nonpregnant adults. Higher or lower doses will be appropriate for some patients.

These guidelines include an explicit method of indicating the order of preference for alternative drug regimens. The recommended order of preference is indicated, where relevant, by a number placed next to each component of a regimen (1 for first preference, 2 for second preference, and so on). Alternatives of equal preference are marked with the same number.

Disclaimer

These guidelines form an acceptable basis for management of patients, but there may be sound clinical reasons for different therapy in individual patients or in specific institutions. The complexity of clinical practice requires that, in all cases, users understand the individual clinical situation, and exercise independent professional judgment when basing therapy on these guidelines. Particularly in complicated situations, these guidelines are not a substitute for seeking appropriate advice.

These guidelines do not include comprehensive drug information, some of which may be important; usually contraindications and precautions for the recommended drugs are not included. Responsible use requires that the prescriber is familiar with these matters.

Independence

Therapeutic Guidelines have been independently prepared and published since the first edition of *Antibiotic Guidelines* in 1978.

Therapeutic Guidelines Limited (TGL) is a not-for-profit independent organisation which is responsible for the production and publication of *Therapeutic Guidelines*. Its funds come solely from sales and subscriptions.

The independence of the *Therapeutic Guidelines* is guaranteed through:

- TGL being independent of government and licensing authorities
- TGL being wholly independent of any form of commercial sponsorship, including the pharmaceutical industry
- the guidelines being free of advertising
- TGL having a strict policy on conflict of interest for directors of TGL and members of the expert groups.

These principles are consistent with those of the International Society of Drug Bulletins, of which TGL is a member.

Process

This text has been prepared by an expert group of experienced clinicians. It represents independent consensus distillation and interpretation of the best available evidence and opinion at the time of publication.

Supporting references are available in the electronic versions of *Therapeutic Guidelines.*

How Therapeutic Guidelines are produced

The aim of TGL is to provide clear, practical, authoritative and succinct therapeutic information for busy health practitioners, for the management of patients with specific conditions.

The guidelines are comprehensive in that they cover all common disorders seen in clinical practice. The information is independent and unbiased and is a distillation of current evidence and opinion. The text is arranged into chapters and sections according to diagnostic entities. Each section gives sufficient surrounding information to orient the reader, followed by succinct and explicit recommendations for therapy.

The guidelines are not primarily meant to instruct, but rather to assist prescribers in ensuring patients receive optimum treatment.

The content of each title is revised by an expert group every two to three years. The iterative cycles are based on response to feedback, and shifts in the evidence base.

The essential principles underlying this process for guideline development stem from the production of the first guidelines in 1978, with the method being both refined and improved over the years.

Choosing the topics

The decision to develop guidelines in an area is determined by the board of TGL. For new areas, the decision is based on one or more of:

- an expressed need by general or specialist practitioners, and/or other groups with interests or involvement in an area
- a perception of possible problems in an area, arising from expressions of dissatisfaction by practitioners or evidence from drug usage data
- a clear problem (eg size of health burden, cost, variations in practice, existence of available evidence) that would be assisted by establishing and promulgating guidelines on what is the most appropriate practice.

The decision to update current titles is based on feedback from clinicians, shifts in the evidence base, changing practice, changing patterns of drug usage or bacterial resistance, and other issues relevant to an area.

Expert group

For most titles, the expert group comprises approximately 12 people—including a chairman, an editor, experts in relevant medical specialties, a general practitioner, a pharmacist and a nurse. Depending on the subject matter, the group may also include experts from other areas, such as physiotherapy and nutrition. Members of expert groups are appointed by the board of TGL. Factors taken into consideration in choosing members include:
- relevant expertise
- scholarship
- constituencies and links to key professional bodies
- ability to work cooperatively
- willingness to challenge conventional thinking
- national representative opinion
- representation from different geographical areas.

Management

The chairman plays a pivotal role in the development of the manuscript as it is that person's responsibility to ensure that the project proceeds harmoniously and according to the set process.

The editor, an employee of TGL, liaises with the chairman and expert group to plan a timetable and to ensure that the manuscript develops effectively, on schedule and within the set budget.

The editor prepares all the papers required for each meeting, including minutes, feedback on the previous edition (when applicable), correspondence regarding content, draft chapters and any other relevant background information.

The editor prepares detailed minutes of each meeting to document the basis for all recommendations, especially those that are new and controversial. The minutes are distributed to all members after each meeting for confirmation.

Inaugural meeting

At the initial meeting of each expert group, explanation and guidance are given to the members on:
- intellectual property
- conflict of interest
- aims and format of the guidelines
- clarification of the scope of the content in light of the target audience
- importance of documentation of evidence to support the recommendations
- desirability of consultation with colleagues expert in the area.

Members of the expert group are asked to declare any interests or relationships they have that might influence their comments, and these are taken into account during ensuing discussions and editing.

Within the subject area, the group decides which, and to what level of detail, specific diagnostic entities need to be covered, taking into consideration the likelihood that a disease will be encountered. In some instances the group may also decide to include advice on some uncommon but serious diseases. Decisions about which entities should be covered may be influenced by feedback from users of an earlier edition.

Members agree on the allocation of tasks, with responsibility for the preparation of initial drafts being taken by individual members.

A schedule for a series of daylong meetings at intervals of approximately eight weeks is planned to allow successive review and discussion of all drafts.

Formulating and revising the guidelines

The starting point for content is what a clinician needs to know to manage a patient with the given condition.

Thus, each section needs to include just sufficient surrounding information to orient the reader, followed by succinct but explicit statements regarding management and recommendations for therapy.

After the inaugural planning meeting, authors prepare initial drafts based on their clinical expertise and the current evidence in the relevant area, with the editor assisting the authors to identify and access relevant supporting information. This may include primary scientific papers, systematic reviews from the Cochrane Collaboration, reviews published in reputable journals and guidelines developed by other credible bodies.

The drafts prepared by the individual authors are circulated to all members of the group well in advance of scheduled meetings to allow ample time for the rest of the group to consider the material before meetings.

Each draft is debated in a face-to-face situation on multiple occasions with discussion becoming successively more exhaustive until every statement in each chapter has been scrutinised, challenged and, if necessary, reworked. Areas in which there is controversy, rapid development or uncertainty are identified and further literature searches undertaken.

The editor liaises with individual authors to document the specific studies used to support the statements and recommendations, and copies of these references are retained on file.

Once the intent of the expert group is clear with respect to specific content, the editor assumes responsibility for the text, reorganising it according to house style and format, and liaising as necessary with authors and the chairman.

The finished manuscript is the result of detailed scrutiny, collaboration and revision, involving a wide range of people and several editing stages. Individual chapters are no longer attributable to any one author. All members of the expert group are responsible for the entire manuscript.

For the preparation of each title, in addition to an inaugural half-day planning meeting, an average of five full-day meetings are required over a period of approximately nine months, with the final meeting being devoted to a final scrutiny of the entire manuscript to ensure all members approve the whole text. The time taken to produce each manuscript, from the inaugural expert group meeting to publication, is approximately 14 months.

Basis of recommendations

The methodology required to develop content for *Therapeutic Guidelines* is different to, and not always entirely compatible with, that used to produce 'reviews or summaries' of the literature. Unlike reviews or summaries where evidence found in the literature determines the basis and scope of a text, the starting point for the development of *Therapeutic Guidelines* is a clinical problem.

The relevance, 'generalisability' and strength of the scientific evidence for the effectiveness of any given treatment are fundamental to the development of the content in *Therapeutic Guidelines*. In clinical areas where there is an abundance of evidence, there can be a reasonably high level of certainty about which treatment(s) should be recommended. But, to make sure that the advice will be helpful for clinicians, the relevant evidence is not only assessed, interpreted, and distilled, but is also contextualised and tailored to the clinical situation, and customised to ensure it is consistent with, or adaptable to, local circumstances.

Decision-making in clinical practice is inherently complex and multifaceted and, in addition to the evidence, other factors need to be considered to ensure the advice is relevant and useful. Examples of such factors include the availability and affordability of the treatment, risk factors and patient characteristics.

'Evidence-rich' areas are in the minority in clinical practice, so a large proportion of the material developed for *Therapeutic Guidelines* is in areas where there is little published evidence.

When the evidence is equivocal, there are sometimes differing but supportable positions. Acceptable alternatives from which prescribers can choose are presented, but ultimately the responsibility for resolving difficulties and producing a clear and unambiguous message based on a considered review of all the evidence and opinion lies with the expert group.

For 'evidence-poor' areas there is necessarily more reliance on expert opinion, and recommendations for therapy are developed based on an assessment of criteria such as the adverse effect profile, long-term safety data, and cost. Using these criteria, older drugs that have been shown to have a reasonable adverse effect profile over a long period of time are often recommended as first-line therapy rather than newer drugs that have a less certain adverse effect profile (particularly in the long term), and are usually more expensive.

If recommendations for treatment were based solely on the scientific evidence, instruments developed by other agencies to assign graded evidence hierarchies to the recommendations could be used. But because factors additional to the evidence are taken into account in the development of the recommendations in *Therapeutic Guidelines*, it is not possible to use these tools.

The approach taken in *Therapeutic Guidelines* to indicate whether a recommendation is based on strong evidence or otherwise is to include explicit statements in the surrounding text.

Major sources of information on which recommendations are based are listed in the electronic versions of *Therapeutic Guidelines*.

External preview and endorsement

Once the manuscript has been finalised and approved by the expert group, it is then circulated for preview by several experts who have been nominated by the chairman or identified by members of the expert group.

Once all feedback has been received, the editor clarifies and collates all comments, and then works with the chairman to ensure all points are considered and any necessary changes are made.

If any substantial change is thought to be required, the expert group is again consulted to ensure that the whole of the final text meets the approval of all members.

Finally, organisations such as The Royal Australian College of General Practitioners, The Royal Australasian College of Physicians, The Society of Hospital Pharmacists of Australia, and Royal College of Nursing Australia, other relevant professional bodies and the National Prescribing Service are invited to endorse the text.

Postpublication evaluation

The evaluation unit of TGL liaises with a network of approximately 160 users (general practitioners, specialists, pharmacists and students) to actively solicit feedback on the guidelines.

Participants in the network are provided with all *Therapeutic Guidelines* free of charge. Staff of TGL visit these users once or twice each year to discuss and record the feedback.

Before any new edition is commenced, accrued feedback on the previous edition is collated and passed on to the expert group for their consideration in the revision of the text.

Users are encouraged to comment about the content or format of the guidelines by completing the form at the back of the book and returning it to TGL, or emailing comments to the evaluation unit <evaluation@tg.com.au>.

BOARD OF DIRECTORS OF TGL

*Associate Professor AR Mant** (chairman)
Woollahra, New South Wales

Dr JS Dowden
Yarralumla, Australian Capital Territory

Professor MR Kidd
Potts Point, New South Wales

Professor JE Marley
New Lambton Heights, New South Wales

Dr ML Mashford
Parkville, Victoria

Mr TK Murphy
Fitzroy, Victoria

Dr JG Primrose†
Farrer, Australian Capital Territory

Dr EE Roughead
Mile End, South Australia

Professor JWG Tiller‡
Melbourne, Victoria

Chief executive officer of TGL
Mrs M Hemming
Fitzroy North, Victoria

Nominees of the following organisations:
* *The Royal Australian College of General Practitioners*
† *Commonwealth Department of Health and Ageing*
‡ *Victorian Medical Postgraduate Foundation Inc.*

Preface

Early in 2005, the National Prescribing Service asked me to attend a meeting with the Australian Dental Association (ADA). As the editor of *Australian Prescriber*, I had been involved in publishing Robin Woods' dental column for many years, so I seemed a likely person to discuss the ADA's plan to publish prescribing guidelines for dental practitioners.

While recognising the importance of Robin Woods' seminal *A Guide to the use of drugs in dentistry*, the ADA saw the need for a small book providing brief practical advice. Preparing practice guidelines is not an easy task, so I suggested that the ADA consider discussing their plans with Therapeutic Guidelines Limited. This company is an independent not-for-profit organisation that has been producing treatment guidelines for Australian medical practitioners since the 1970s. Titles such as *Therapeutic Guidelines: Antibiotic* are internationally recognised for their usefulness to prescribers. There was therefore a great potential for the ADA to tap into the wealth of information that had already been prepared by Therapeutic Guidelines.

The discussions between the ADA and Therapeutic Guidelines were fruitful, and an agreement was reached for Therapeutic Guidelines to assist the ADA in preparing guidelines for dental practitioners. Later in 2005, I had the honour of being invited to chair the group preparing the guidelines, and in August 2005 the expert group met for the first time.

There have been seven meetings of the expert group, but much of the work has been done between the meetings. Each chapter began as a draft based on clinical evidence and with reference to previously published guidelines. These drafts were then critically reviewed and discussed by the expert group. For some topics, this process has been repeated several times until we have agreed on practical recommendations. To further enhance the quality of the guidelines, many chapters have been sent for external peer review by Australian and international experts. The resultant publication is therefore the culmination of many hours of work by many people.

The aim of the guidelines has always been to assist general dental practitioners in their day-to-day practice. These guidelines provide sound advice that will help them deal with most situations where a prescription may be required. The guidelines may also be of assistance to other health professionals, particularly those working in remote areas, if they are consulted by patients with dental problems. In some cases nondrug treatment is recommended rather than a prescription. As the guidelines do not cover every aspect of advanced dental practice, specialist referral is sometimes indicated.

These guidelines are not a book of rules to limit practice. They have no legal standing, but represent a consensus view based on the available evidence that I hope points the way towards 'best practice'.

The real test for these guidelines will be their usefulness in practice. I therefore encourage readers to forward their comments about this publication. These comments will be of great help for future editions.

While looking to the future, I must thank the expert group for their perseverance and enthusiasm in preparing this first edition. John Matthews of the ADA has been particularly helpful in promoting the project, and Jill Pope of Therapeutic Guidelines has done a wonderful job of managing the writing process.

As a consumer of dental treatment I have already found the guidelines to be invaluable. I hope they work for you too!

Dr John S Dowden
Chairman
Expert Group for *Therapeutic Guidelines: Oral and Dental*
January 2007

Principles of diagnosis and prescribing

There are a number of general principles that must be followed before treating any disease (see Box 1). The first, and most important, is to identify the disease and its cause—that is, to make a diagnosis. The second principle is to remove the cause so the disease cannot recur. Once these two aspects have been followed, the other general principles should be followed in sequence; these are removing the effect(s) of the disease, restoring the tissues to their normal function, monitoring the healing, observing the stability of the area over time, and preventing recurrence of the disease.

The process of making a diagnosis should be considered an 'information gathering exercise'. The necessary information can be obtained by taking a thorough history, doing a complete clinical examination and performing the appropriate diagnostic tests. Once the information has been gathered, the clinician should collate it and decide on the diagnosis. This process requires that the dental clinician has a thorough working knowledge of the various disease processes that may affect the oral and dental tissues and surrounding structures, plus a thorough knowledge of the various systemic diseases that may manifest in the mouth.

> **Box 1. General principles of treating disease**
>
> Identify the disease and its cause.
>
> Remove the cause.
>
> Remove the effect of the disease.
>
> Restore the tissues to their normal function.
>
> Monitor the healing.
>
> Observe the stability of the area over time.
>
> Prevent recurrence of the disease.

HISTORY

The first stage of taking a history should be to **determine the patient's presenting complaint** or their reason for attending the dental surgery. This allows the clinician to focus on the particular problem of concern to the patient, so the patient can be managed effectively and efficiently, and the appropriate treatment can be provided.

The **medical history** should then follow, as this may provide information essential to the diagnosis of the presenting problem, or it may dictate that modifications to the management of the patient are required. The medical history should include allergies—and to what—and medications being taken (including over-the-counter, complementary and alternative medicines). The medical history should be checked periodically, as both the health status and the medications being taken may change over time.

The **dental history** should include an overview of the patient's previous dental problems and treatment, and a detailed history of the presenting condition. While listening to the patient's outline of the presenting problem, the clinician should begin to formulate a *provisional* diagnosis—the clinician should think of several potential diagnoses (ie differential diagnoses), and then ask specific questions to provide more information to narrow the possible range of diseases and so form the provisional diagnosis. 'Open-ended' questions should be asked rather than 'leading' questions, as the latter may be answered by the patient in the way that they 'think' the clinician wants them to answer (eg the clinician should ask the patient what particular things cause the pain, rather than asking if hot and cold drinks cause the pain).

EXAMINATION AND INVESTIGATIONS

The clinician should form a provisional diagnosis before starting the clinical examination, so the examination and diagnostic tests can be targeted towards confirming the diagnosis and identifying which tooth or other tissues are involved. It is not always necessary to perform every possible diagnostic test; clinicians must choose tests that are relevant to the presenting complaint. Ideally, for most diseases, there should be at least two signs or symptoms present to indicate the disease process. If there is any doubt, either the clinician should defer treatment (if the pain is not severe) until the diagnosis becomes clear, or the patient should be referred for diagnosis and treatment by a specialist. Irreversible treatment should never be commenced until a definitive diagnosis has been established, because the diagnosis determines the treatment required. The approach of 'let's try this and see what happens' should be avoided, as it may lead to incorrect and/or inappropriate treatment being provided, and it may mask important signs or symptoms that would help to establish a diagnosis.

Specific tests may be required to provide further information as part of the diagnostic process. Such tests should *not* be considered as 'special tests' but as routine or required tests for the specific condition being considered (eg pulp sensibility tests and periapical radiographs are required for the diagnosis of pulp and periapical diseases; probing of periodontal pockets is essential for periodontal disease; blood tests may be required for some mucosal disorders; a biopsy may be required for some lesions). It is important that the appropriate diagnostic tests and procedures for the suspected condition are utilised.

The diagnosis of any disease is incomplete if the cause of the disease has not been determined. The cause may be simple (eg dental caries as a cause for pulp disease), or complex (eg a medical syndrome or disease); complex conditions may require other management in addition to dental treatment. It is essential to identify the cause(s) of the disease, because removing the cause(s) is an integral part (and usually the first stage) of managing the disease. If the cause is not removed, full or rapid recovery from the presenting condition may not occur, and the presenting condition may merely be converted from an acute and painful condition to a chronic state with reduced or no symptoms—but with the disease still present and slowly progressing.

Good clinical records should be kept—with the diagnosis *recorded*. Box 2 shows the aspects of the examination and diagnosis that should be included in the records.

Box 2. Aspects of the examination and diagnosis that should be included in clinical records

A description of the patient's presenting complaint

The medical and dental histories (including medications)

The clinical findings

The results of all tests performed

A radiographic report

The diagnosis

The cause

A management plan including specific treatment to be provided

Details of all discussions with, and advice given to, the patient

MANAGEMENT

There is a distinction between 'management' and 'treatment'. **Management** can be defined as 'the act, art and manner of handling a situation'; it includes skilful, careful and tactful treatment. **Treatment** is defined as 'a systematic course of medical or surgical care'. These definitions indicate that management includes treatment, but management also includes the overall handling of the patient and their problems in a sensitive manner. It is preferable for clinicians to 'manage' the patient and their problems rather than just 'treating' them.

Drugs should not be prescribed without having a definitive diagnosis, otherwise an inappropriate drug or an incorrect dose regimen may be used. In addition, the drug may mask the symptoms, which makes further examination and diagnosis even more difficult. The concept of prescribing a drug 'to see if it helps' or 'just in case' should be avoided since it indicates that an accurate and definitive diagnosis has not been made. There is a real risk of adverse effects with every drug, and therefore drugs should only be prescribed if there is likely to be a demonstrable benefit. If a drug is not required, it should not be used and then the risk is nonexistent.

Drugs should not be prescribed as the sole means of managing most dental and oral problems. Most conditions that lead a patient to visit their dental practitioner also require some form of active dental (or oral) treatment, and such treatment is usually the most effective and efficient means of managing most dental emergencies or pain problems. When considering the management of all dental (and most oral) conditions, the principle of the '3 Ds' should be remembered:

- **D**iagnosis—The disease and its cause must always be determined first.
- **D**ental treatment—Once the diagnosis has been determined, then the appropriate dental treatment should be provided; this includes removing the cause(s) of the disease.
- **D**rugs—The final consideration is whether any drugs are required; this decision should be deferred until the response to the dental treatment has been reviewed.

If these principles are followed by clinicians, the drugs commonly used in dentistry (antibiotics, analgesics and anti-inflammatory agents) can often be avoided (or at least minimised); this means they are likely to be more effective when they are actually required. They are also far more likely to be effective since the cause of the disease has been removed and the appropriate dental treatment has been initiated.

Prescriptions and prescription-writing

If prescribers have a clear understanding of both the importance of prescribing appropriately and also the processes involved, they can prescribe rationally and independently, and without fear of coercion. Inappropriate prescribing can lead to ineffective and unsafe treatment; it can exacerbate or prolong illness; it can cause distress or harm to patients; and it can be more costly than prescribing appropriately.

It has been estimated that approximately 140 000 Australians are hospitalised annually because of adverse reactions to prescription medicines. Many more people suffer adverse drug reactions without needing hospitalisation. Most adverse reactions are preventable, by clinicians taking an appropriate history and prescribing rationally.

Treatment of any sort needs to be effective, safe and affordable. Where the treatment involves the use of drugs, the prescriber must use up-to-date knowledge to choose the best option for treatment for the particular patient and their specific problem. Prescribing is part of a logical deductive process based on comprehensive and objective information. The patient should be involved as a partner in management decisions, and the option of not using drug treatment should always be considered. Most conditions that lead a patient to visit their dental practitioner require some form of active dental (or oral) treatment, and drugs are usually only needed *in addition to* other treatments.

THE PROCESS OF RATIONAL TREATMENT

The process of rational treatment involves:
- defining the problem
- specifying the therapeutic objective (eg pain relief, infection prevention, treatment)
- choosing the treatment. In dentistry, drugs are usually an adjunct to physical treatment. Choice is based on
  - efficacy
  - safety
  - suitability (eg adherence [compliance] issues, coexisting conditions for this particular patient, drug formulation)
  - cost.

Before commencing treatment, it is essential that a prescriber has a full medical and medication history of the patient; this includes:
- age and weight
- allergies
- a history of adverse drug reactions
- any medical condition the patient is suffering from
- any medications that the patient is taking (from any source; ie prescription drugs, over-the-counter medicines, complementary and alternative medicines, alcohol and other 'recreational' drugs).

Starting treatment involves:
- giving the patient clear instructions and information about both the condition and the reasons for the treatment
- doing appropriate dental or oral treatment
- if required, writing an appropriate and accurate prescription.

Monitoring progress involves:
- reviewing the patient
- deciding whether to stop, continue or change the treatment
- deciding whether ongoing medication is appropriate.

Prescribers need to be confident in their ability to evaluate information about drugs and to determine their therapeutic value. Confidence is enhanced by having a list of preferred drugs and becoming thoroughly familiar with their use. New and expensive drugs should be critically evaluated before they are used in the place of established treatments.

PATIENT FACTORS

The use of any drug must reflect the therapeutic need of the patient. It is important to identify if the patient is in a high-risk group (eg older persons, children, those who are pregnant, those with kidney or liver disease or any other chronic condition), and if they are taking medications (including nonprescription medications).

Patients may demand particular drugs, or the prescriber may presume they are requesting certain drugs. Good communication helps avoid presumed patient demands, and good prescribing habits help counter patient demands caused by advertising, addiction, or unrealistic expectations.

Always consider alternatives to drug treatment and give the patient the reasons why the alternative may be in their best interests.

PRINCIPLES OF PRESCRIBING

Base decisions on evidence-based practice.

Be aware of risk and benefits (eg the risk of an orthopaedic implant becoming infected once it is established is approximately 0.03%, whereas the risk of an adverse reaction to antibiotics is around 3%).

Follow medical prescribing principles, which, for acute pain and infection, generally advocate rapidly reaching satisfactory blood levels and then using small incremental doses as required.

Overprescribing and underprescribing

It is important that the duration of treatment, the dose, and the quantity of drugs prescribed are accurate.

Overprescribing is wasteful, can cause unnecessary adverse effects, and increases the opportunities for overdoses; also, some drugs are addictive if overused.

Underprescribing is also wasteful, and is potentially harmful. It can result in ineffective treatment, and the patient may need a different and more expensive treatment later.

THE PRESCRIPTION

A prescription is a legal document; it must be a precise written instruction from a prescriber (medical practitioner, dental practitioner, veterinary surgeon, some optometrists, some podiatrists and, in some states, nurse practitioners) to a pharmacist on behalf of a patient. Who may write prescriptions and how they should be written are outlined in the appropriate state legislation (Acts and Regulations) (see pp.11–12).

Prescribers should always write the drug names in full. The instructions must be written with full English words (not in Latin or in any form of abbreviation). Instructions should clearly state how the prescriber wishes the patient to use the medication. It is *not* appropriate to write 'take as directed', because a significant number of patients forget a prescriber's verbal instructions within a few minutes.

The prescriber has a duty of care to provide a prescription that is *legible*; this reduces the potential for errors in treatment. An illegible prescription can constitute professional negligence. Computer-generated prescriptions are generally more legible than those that are handwritten. However, just because a prescription is computer-generated, it does not mean that an error has not occurred. The principle to be followed is one of constant checking.

Essential information required for a legal prescription written by a dental practitioner comprises:
- prescriber's name, address and telephone number
- patient's full name (given and family names) and address
- date the prescription is written
- drug name (preferably generic or approved name)
- drug strength (eg 250 mg, 500 mg)
- drug form (eg tablet, capsule or mixture)
- quantity of drug
- drug dose, manner of administration, frequency, and duration of treatment (if necessary)
- clear instructions for the patient (in English)
- any further instructions necessary for the pharmacist
- the words 'for dental treatment only'
- signature of the prescriber—handwritten.

If the prescription is for an item included in the Pharmaceutical Benefit Scheme (PBS), the dental practitioner's unique prescriber number must be on the prescription. (PBS prescription pads are available from Medicare Australia.) Figure 1 has an example of the format required for a legal prescription written by a dentist.

Points to note when writing a prescription are as follows:
- Make the prescription as tamper-proof (unalterable) as possible and use indelible ink.
- Do not write prescriptions for more than one person on the same form.
- It may be useful to include the patient's date of birth.
- Write drug names in full.
- Use standard language for instruction.
- Do *not* use abbreviations or Latin terms.
- Avoid using decimal points, if possible (eg write quantities less than 1 gram as milligrams, and quantities less than 1 milligram as micrograms).
- If using a decimal point put a '0' in front of the point (eg not '.5' but '0.5').
- Do *not* abbreviate microgram, nanogram, international or unit.
- Use millilitres (mL), not cubic centimetres.
- Limit the number of items on a prescription to two or, at the most, three.
- Use computer-generated prescriptions (if possible).

Figure 1. Example of the format required for a legal prescription

```
                                          Dr J Smith BDSc
                                                  Address
                                         Telephone number
                                    PBS prescribing number

Patient's Medicare number   ................................................
Patient's name              Ms Jane Citizen
Patient's address           ................................................



        Rx

            Phenoxymethylpenicillin 500 mg capsules

            25

            Take 1 capsule 4 times a day at 6-hourly intervals




                              Signature................................
                              Date.....................................

                        For dental treatment only
```

- If using trade or brand names, ensure that you know what the actual approved or generic substance is.
- If any space is left unused, put a line across the area to prevent the addition of items.

Prescribers and pharmacists have complementary roles in ensuring optimum patient outcomes. This is enhanced by mutual respect for each other's skills.

THE PRESCRIPTION AND THE PATIENT

When prescribing drugs, give the patient specific information about the drug, including:
- the effects of the drug and why it is needed
- possible adverse effects and what to do if they occur
- instructions on how to take the drug
- warnings (eg possible interactions, maximum dose)
- when to return for review
- permission to ring you if concerned about any issues.

People often do not remember the details or instructions that they are given during a consultation, so it is desirable to give written instructions as well. Consumer medication information (CMI) leaflets written by pharmaceutical companies to reflect approved product information are available from pharmacies and some prescribing software packages, and should be given to patients.

SOURCES OF DRUG INFORMATION

Recommended sources of drug information include the following books, journals and websites.

Journals and bulletins
- *Australian Dental Journal* (ADJ)—see 'Medications in dentistry supplement' in December 2005 edition
- *Australian Prescriber* <www.australianprescriber.com>

Books
- *Australian Medicines Handbook* (AMH)—an annual publication (print and CD-ROM) including a section on prescription-writing as well as evidence-based information about drugs
- *Therapeutic Guidelines* (*Analgesic, Antibiotic, Cardiovascular, Dermatology, Endocrinology, Gastrointestinal, Neurology, Psychotropic, Palliative Care, Respiratory, Rheumatology, Management Guidelines: Developmental Disability* [and *eTG complete* and *miniTG*])
- *MIMS Annual* and *MIMS* bi-monthly (can be accessed via the Australian Dental Association website <http://www.ada.org.au>)
- *Drug interaction facts* (Tatro DS, editor. St Louis: Facts and comparisons [hard copy and CD, updated 3-monthly]). This is an excellent resource on drug interactions
- Any recent textbook on clinical pharmacology

AMH and *MIMS* have sections on drug–drug interactions that a prescribing dental practitioner can consult if a patient is already taking medications from a different prescriber.

Websites
- Pharmaceutical Benefits Scheme (PBS) website <http://www.health.gov.au/pbs>
- Australian Dental Association website <http://www.ada.org.au>
- Pharmacist-relevant website <http://auspharmacist.net.au/>, which has links to a large number of sites with drug information
- National Prescribing Service (NPS) <http://www.nps.org.au>

LEGISLATION ABOUT PRESCRIPTIONS AND PRESCRIBING

Below is a list of legislation pertaining to prescriptions and prescribing in each of the states and territories. Overall, there are no significant differences in the requirements for what constitutes a legal prescription, but there are some minor differences. If dental practitioners are in doubt, they should consult the appropriate legislation for their state or territory.

The Schedule of Pharmaceutical Benefits lists a number of medicines that are subsidised by the Pharmaceutical Benefits Scheme (PBS) if prescribed by a dentist. Dentists may prescribe any 'prescription-only' medicine provided it is for dental treatment of a patient under their care.

> ***Additional caution should be exercised when prescribing drugs of dependence.***

Dentists may prescribe any drug of dependence (in most states and territories) for a patient under their care provided they do so in accordance with legal requirements, and have taken all reasonable steps to ascertain the identity of that person and to ensure that a therapeutic need exists, and the drug is required for *dental* treatment.

Dentists may not order repeat prescriptions.

Relevant regulations

The following are the relevant Acts and Regulations in each state and territory. They can be accessed via the ADA website <http://www.ada.org.au>.

Australian Capital Territory
Drugs of Dependence Act 1989
Drugs of Dependence Regulation 2005

Poisons and Drug Act 1978
Poisons and Drug Regulation 1993

Poisons Act 1933
Poisons Regulation 1933

New South Wales
Poisons and Therapeutic Goods Act 1966
Poisons and Therapeutic Goods Regulation 2002

Northern Territory
Poisons and Dangerous Drugs Act
Poisons and Dangerous Drugs Regulations

Therapeutic Goods and Cosmetics Act

Queensland
Health Act 1937
Health (Drugs and Poisons) Regulation 1996

South Australia
Controlled Substances Act 1984
Controlled Substances Regulations 1996

Tasmania
Poisons Act 1971
Poisons Regulations 2002

Victoria
Drugs, Poisons and Controlled Substances Act 1981
Drugs, Poisons and Controlled Substances Regulations 2006

Western Australia
Poisons Act 1964
Poisons Regulations 1965

Getting to know your drugs

Practitioners must know both the effects and the adverse effects of the drugs they prescribe. Practitioners should choose drugs they are familiar with, and use appropriate sources of drug information (see p.10 for some resources). When practitioners are prescribing drugs and analysing potential drug interactions, they must be aware of concurrent drug use, including over-the-counter and complementary medicines, as well as the current medical condition of the patient.

ANTIMICROBIALS

General considerations

The problems posed by pathogenic organisms resistant to antimicrobial drugs (both established and new) are increasing globally. Adherence to the principles of antimicrobial use (see Box 3, p.14) is increasingly important. Refer to *Therapeutic Guidelines: Antibiotic* for antimicrobial agents not covered in these guidelines.

> ***Restraint in the use of all antimicrobials is the best way to ensure their continuing efficacy.***

Most conditions requiring antimicrobial treatment can be managed using established drugs. This is reflected in the recommendations made in these guidelines.

> ***It must be determined whether an antimicrobial drug is actually needed. Most viral and minor bacterial diseases are self-limiting and do not benefit from the use of antimicrobials.***

Unnecessary prescription of antimicrobials exposes patients to adverse drug effects, is costly, and helps create conditions that favour the proliferation of resistant organisms in the patient and the community. Before prescribing an antimicrobial, the question needs to be asked, 'Is this really necessary for this patient?' When prescribing an antibiotic, a dental practitioner might like to consider the principles embodied in the mnemonic for the antibiotic creed, MIND ME (see Box 4, p.14).

Box 3. Principles of use of antibiotics*

General

Use antibiotics only where the benefits are scientifically demonstrable and substantial.

Use the narrowest spectrum antimicrobial to treat the known or likely pathogen(s).

Use single drugs unless it has been proven that combination therapy is required to ensure efficacy or to reduce the selection of clinically significant resistance.

Use a dose that is high enough to ensure efficacy and minimise the risk of resistance selection.

Use a dose that is low enough to minimise risk of dose-related toxicity.

Therapy

Base the choice of therapy on either known common pathogens in the condition and their current resistance patterns (empirical therapy) or culture and susceptibility test results (directed therapy).

Duration of use should be as short as possible, and should not exceed 7 days[†] unless there is proof that this duration is inadequate.

Prophylaxis

Base choice of antimicrobial on known or likely target pathogen(s).

Duration should be as short as possible. A single dose of antibiotic is recommended for surgical prophylaxis if required for dental procedures.

---

* Modified from: The use of antibiotics in food-producing animals: antibiotic-resistant bacteria in animals and humans. Report of the Joint Expert Advisory Committee on Antibiotic Resistance (JETACAR). Canberra: Commonwealth Department of Health and Aged Care and Commonwealth Department of Agriculture, Fisheries and Forestry; 1999. p.164. <http://www.health.gov.au/internet/wcms/Publishing.nsf/Content/health-pubs-jetacar-cnt.htm>.
[†] For most odontogenic infections, 5 days is sufficient.

Box 4. The antibiotic creed

M	Microbiology guides therapy wherever possible
I	Indications should be evidence-based
N	Narrowest spectrum required
D	Dosage appropriate to the site and type of infection
M	Minimise duration of therapy
E	Ensure monotherapy in most situations

Some groups of antimicrobial drugs used in dentistry, and examples of each group, are shown in Table 1 (p.16).

Potential problems with antibiotics

Resistance

Antimicrobial resistance is increasing in many pathogens. Problem organisms include *Streptococcus pneumoniae*, methicillin-resistant *Staphylococcus aureus* (MRSA), vancomycin-resistant enterococci (VRE), strains of *Klebsiella* and *Escherichia coli* with extended-spectrum cephalosporin resistance, and multiresistant *Acinetobacter* and *Pseudomonas aeruginosa*. Emergence of resistance to reserve antibiotics such as the fluoroquinolones, the carbapenems and vancomycin is also of concern. Antibiotic use is one of the pressures that increases resistance. Appropriate antibiotic use will delay the emergence of resistance and minimise resistance prevalence after it has emerged. There is strong evidence that methicillin-resistant *Staphylococcus aureus* (MRSA) is becoming more common in the community. The Centers for Disease Control and Prevention website has useful information on how to prevent antimicrobial resistance in health care settings—see <http://www.cdc.gov/drugresistance/healthcare/patients.htm>.

Hypersensitivity (allergy)

Antibiotic hypersensitivity is common, and most frequently involves beta lactams (eg phenoxymethylpenicillin, cephalexin). While many nonspecific reactions are labelled as 'allergic', true type I (IgE-mediated) antibiotic hypersensitivity is strongly suggested by the development of urticaria, angioedema, bronchospasm, or anaphylaxis (with objectively demonstrated hypotension, hypoxia or tryptase elevation) within one hour of drug administration. Some instances of 'pseudo-allergy' (eg anaphylactoid responses to vancomycin infusions, such as 'red-man syndrome') involve direct release of vasoactive mediators by non-IgE mechanisms.

Drug allergy is more commonly seen with certain infections, particularly with HIV and Epstein-Barr virus infections, and allergic reactions are more likely to be severe in individuals receiving beta-blocker therapy.

Diagnosis of hypersensitivity

Antibiotic hypersensitivity is usually diagnosed on the basis of clinical history, with oral challenging judiciously employed where skin tests (if performed) are negative, or in circumstances where alternative drugs

Table 1. Antimicrobial drugs used in dentistry

	Examples
Antibacterial drugs	
beta lactams	
penicillins	
narrow-spectrum penicillins	benzylpenicillin, phenoxymethylpenicillin
narrow-spectrum penicillins with antistaphylococcal activity	dicloxacillin, flucloxacillin, methicillin
moderate-spectrum penicillins	amoxycillin, ampicillin
broad-spectrum penicillins (beta-lactamase–inhibitor combinations)	amoxycillin+clavulanate
broad-spectrum penicillins with antipseudomonal activity	piperacillin, ticarcillin
cephalosporins	
moderate-spectrum cephalosporins	cephalexin, cephalothin, cephazolin
moderate-spectrum cephalosporins with anti-*Haemophilus* activity	cefaclor, cefuroxime
moderate-spectrum cephalosporins with antianaerobic activity	cefoxitin
broad-spectrum cephalosporins	cefotaxime, ceftriaxone
broad-spectrum cephalosporins with antipseudomonal activity	cefepime, ceftazidime
carbapenems	imipenem, meropenem
glycopeptides	vancomycin, teicoplanin
lincosamides	clindamycin, lincomycin
macrolides	clarithromycin, erythromycin, roxithromycin
nitroimidazoles	metronidazole, tinidazole
tetracyclines	doxycycline, tetracycline
Antifungal drugs	
azoles	clotrimazole, ketoconazole, miconazole
polyenes	amphotericin, nystatin

continued next page

Table 1. Antimicrobial drugs used in dentistry (cont.)

	Examples
Antiviral drugs	
guanine analogues	aciclovir, famciclovir, valaciclovir
thymidine analogue	idoxuridine

are clearly inferior. The confirmation of antibiotic hypersensitivity is difficult, as no currently available skin or blood test offers 100% negative predictive value for drug allergy.

Penicillin hypersensitivity

Between 1% and 10% of beta-lactam courses result in manifestations interpreted as being due to hypersensitivity. Most reactions are late, non–IgE-mediated and involve skin rash. Other later manifestations include fever, haemolysis and serum sickness–like reactions. The minority of reactions are immediate hypersensitivity reactions. Anaphylactic responses to penicillin occur approximately once every 10 000 courses administered, with 10% of these reactions being fatal. Most of these reactions occur in people without a history of prior penicillin allergy. Notwithstanding this, a detailed history of a reaction to a beta lactam should always be sought before a course of a penicillin is commenced.

> *A history of an immediate hypersensitivity reaction (urticaria, angioedema, bronchospasm, or anaphylaxis within one hour of drug administration) or other life-threatening reactions (eg Stevens-Johnson syndrome) contraindicates further exposure to penicillin and other beta lactams.*

Rashes, particularly with amoxy/ampicillin, are much less predictive of future reactions, and repeat exposure to beta-lactam drugs is not necessarily contraindicated.

Between 3% and 10% of patients hypersensitive to penicillins exhibit cross-reactivity with cephalosporins and carbapenems.

A patient with a known beta-lactam hypersensitivity should be encouraged to wear an alert bracelet or necklace containing this information.

Antibiotic-associated diarrhoea

Diarrhoea is an adverse effect of many antibiotics. In patients with severe diarrhoea, pseudomembranous colitis can occur. The most frequently implicated drugs causing antibiotic-associated diarrhoea are lincosamides (clindamycin, lincomycin), cephalosporins and ampicillin. Antibiotics that are implicated less frequently are other penicillins, erythromycin, sulfamethoxazole+trimethoprim and sulfasalazine.

In most cases of antibiotic-associated diarrhoea, no pathogen is identified. If the diarrhoea requires intervention, the first step is to cease treatment, if possible, with any antibiotic likely to be causing the symptoms.

Antibiotics and interactions with oral contraceptives

There is a small risk of interactions between oral contraceptives and common antimicrobials used in dentistry. The general recommendation is that women who have had a broad-spectrum antibiotic prescribed should continue with their oral contraception as well as use an alternative method of contraception while taking the antibiotics and for seven days after completing the course of treatment.

Antimicrobial choice

When an antimicrobial drug is indicated, the prescriber should base the choice on factors such as:
- spectrum of activity in relation to the known or suspected causative organism(s)
- safety of drug (including adverse reactions and interactions)
- previous clinical experience
- cost
- potential for selection of resistant organisms
- associated risk of superinfection
- patient factors.

The relative importance of each of these factors will be influenced by the severity of the illness and whether the drug is to be used for prophylaxis, empirical therapy or directed therapy.

> ***A history of hypersensitivity or other adverse response to the drug under consideration should be sought and taken into account.***

Knowledge of a previous adverse drug reaction may prevent the inadvertent administration of an antimicrobial drug to which the patient is allergic. Failure to take an adequate history can have serious and sometimes fatal consequences.

Additional care must be taken in the elderly, as the pharmacokinetic or toxicodynamic profiles may be altered. Renal or hepatic impairment may require adjustment of the dose or dosing interval. Where therapy is to be self-administered, consider the complexity of the dosage regimen, particularly for those on multiple therapies or with cognitive impairment. See also Box 3 (p.14) for principles of antibiotic use.

The choice of therapy should be based on either known common pathogens in the condition and their current resistance patterns (empirical therapy), or culture and susceptibility test results (directed therapy).

Empirical therapy

Therapy is empirical when it is based on known common pathogens in the condition and their current resistance patterns. Prescribers should base empirical antimicrobial therapy on local epidemiological data, and on potential pathogens and their patterns of antimicrobial susceptibility. Once commenced, continue antimicrobials for at least 48 hours. Where appropriate, obtain specimens for Gram stain, culture and susceptibility testing before commencing antimicrobial therapy. A Gram stain (eg of pus) or direct antigen detection methods may allow specific (directed) therapy to be commenced even before the pathogen has been cultured.

Directed therapy

Therapy is directed when it is based on culture and susceptibility test results. It is important to review the empirical regimen when culture results have identified the organisms present and their susceptibility to antimicrobial drugs (remembering that organisms found to be present may not necessarily be responsible for the clinical condition). Laboratory data must be interpreted in the context of the overall clinical picture. The natural resolution of a bacterial infection may result from host defences, despite laboratory-reported resistance. Antimicrobial therapy directed at specific organisms should include the most effective, least toxic, narrowest spectrum drug available. This reduces the problems associated with broad-spectrum therapy (ie selection of and superinfection with resistant microorganisms), and usually is the most cost-effective.

Combination therapy

Avoid antimicrobial combinations, unless indicated to:
- broaden the antibacterial spectrum (eg empirical therapy of suspected mixed infections, such as spreading neck infections)
- achieve synergy that is known to improve outcomes (eg enterococcal endocarditis)
- prevent the emergence of resistant microorganisms (eg therapy of tuberculosis).

Modes of delivery

Oral and parenteral therapy

Compared with oral administration, parenteral use of antimicrobials has several disadvantages, including greater risk of serious adverse events (including line-associated sepsis), higher drug product cost, additional cost of equipment, and additional time and expertise needed for administration.

Oral therapy should be used in preference to parenteral therapy unless:
- oral administration is not tolerated or is not possible (eg swallowing difficulties)
- gastrointestinal absorption is an obvious problem (eg vomiting, severe diarrhoea, gastrointestinal disease), or a potential problem that may accentuate poor bioavailability of an oral antimicrobial
- an oral antimicrobial with a suitable spectrum of activity is unavailable
- high doses are required to achieve effective concentrations at the site of infection (eg for endocarditis, meningitis, osteomyelitis, septic arthritis) and are not readily achievable by oral administration
- urgent treatment is required due to severe and rapidly progressing illness
- the patient is unlikely to adhere to oral treatment.

If **parenteral administration** (eg intravenous, intramuscular, subcutaneous) is used, seek appropriate health practitioner assistance. Patients requiring parenteral administration may need to be hospitalised. Reassess the need for parenteral antibiotics daily, and convert to oral therapy as soon as possible.

Topical therapy

It is important to restrict topical antimicrobial therapy to a few proven indications (eg miconazole for oral candidosis). In general, antimicrobials recommended for topical use should not be from classes of antimicrobials used for systemic therapy.

Intradental therapy

Antibiotics may be used within the root canal system of teeth. Commercial preparations containing antibiotics usually also contain a corticosteroid.

These preparations are used to manage intracanal infections and apical periodontitis, and to reduce inflammatory root resorption.

Duration of therapy

To minimise the development of antibiotic resistance, it is important to limit the duration of therapy. In most bacterial infections, the optimal duration of therapy is not well defined. For most odontogenic infections, five days is sufficient.

> *If dental treatment has been provided (as it should be), generally only a short course is required if an antibiotic is indicated.*

Antibacterial drugs

Most of the antibacterial drugs listed below are subsidised by the Pharmaceutical Benefits Scheme. However, dentists are not precluded from prescribing any drug approved by the Therapeutic Goods Administration (TGA), provided the drug is prescribed as part of the dental treatment for a patient that the dental practitioner has established (by examination) needs the drug.

Beta lactams

The beta lactams (eg cephalosporins and penicillins) are structurally related and share bactericidal activity primarily directed at the bacterial cell wall. Most beta lactams are relatively safe, except in patients who are hypersensitive to them. The combination of beta lactams with an inhibitor of beta-lactamase has important applications (see 'Broad-spectrum penicillins [beta-lactamase–inhibitor combinations]', p.23). Examples of beta lactams and their categories are shown in Table 1 (p.16).

Adverse effects: The most serious adverse effects of beta lactams are hypersensitivity (allergy) (see p.15), and diarrhoea (see p.17). The most common adverse effects are gastrointestinal, and generally tend to be mild and self-limiting.

Precautions: The major problem associated with beta lactams is the likelihood of bacteria developing resistance to antibiotics. (See p.15 for development of antibiotic resistance.)

Interactions: The major interaction of beta lactams is with probenecid (a uricosuric agent), which competes with beta lactams for active secretion, giving rise to significantly increased blood levels of beta-lactam antibiotics. This interaction is used deliberately to increase plasma levels of beta lactams where such high levels are required.

Penicillins

Adverse effects: The most common adverse effects of the penicillins are nausea, diarrhoea, rash, urticaria, pain and inflammation (at the injection site), and superinfection (after prolonged treatment and/or with broad-spectrum penicillins). See also p.15 for hypersensitivity and for antibiotic resistance, and p.17 for antibiotic-associated diarrhoea.

Narrow-spectrum penicillins

Narrow-spectrum penicillins are active mainly against Gram-positive organisms, and they are inactivated by beta-lactamases.

For adverse effects, precautions and interactions, see above and p.21.

Phenoxymethylpenicillin (penicillin V) is acid-stable, so it can be given orally, although food impairs absorption; hence it should be taken one hour before a meal or two hours after eating. It is intrinsically less active than benzylpenicillin. It is the drug of first choice in odontogenic infections due to its narrow (and appropriate) spectrum of activity. It has fewer gastrointestinal problems than amoxycillin and is less likely to cause a rash.

Benzylpenicillin (penicillin G) is administered parenterally and is the treatment of choice for susceptible infections if parenteral treatment is warranted.

Narrow-spectrum penicillins with antistaphylococcal activity

Dicloxacillin and **flucloxacillin** are stable to beta-lactamase produced by staphylococci. They are reliably absorbed by the oral route; however, food reduces absorption and they are best taken half to one hour before food. Flucloxacillin and dicloxacillin are generally well tolerated, but are occasionally associated with cholestatic jaundice, particularly in older patients on prolonged therapy. They are rarely indicated in general dental practice.

For adverse effects, precautions and interactions, see above and p.21.

Moderate-spectrum penicillins

The aminopenicillins, **amoxycillin** and **ampicillin**, have good activity against some Gram-negative organisms (eg *Escherichia coli*, *Haemophilus influenzae*), but they are destroyed by beta-lactamase–producing strains. They are drugs of choice for enterococcal infections. Amoxycillin is better absorbed orally than ampicillin, is not affected significantly by food, and requires fewer oral doses per day. When administered parenterally they are equivalent. In these guidelines, amoxy/ampicillin refers to amoxycillin or ampicillin.

For adverse effects and precautions, see p.21 and p.22.

Interactions: In addition to the interactions shown on p.21, amoxycillin and ampicillin, when given to a patient who is taking allopurinol (used in the prevention of gout), increase the likelihood of the patient developing a rash.

Broad-spectrum penicillins (beta-lactamase–inhibitor combinations)

The beta-lactamase inhibitor **clavulanate** inhibits the enzymes produced by *Staphylococcus aureus* and *Bacteroides fragilis* and also the beta-lactamase enzymes found in *Escherichia coli*, *Klebsiella* species, *Neisseria gonorrhoeae* and *Haemophilus influenzae*. The drug possesses little inherent antibacterial activity, but significantly extends the spectrum of activity of amoxycillin when given with it. The combination should be reserved for the treatment of infections caused by organisms in which resistance to the beta lactam is due to enzymes that the beta-lactamase inhibitor is able to inhibit.

Adverse effects: Amoxycillin+clavulanate can cause diarrhoea and hepatotoxicity, which occur more frequently than with amoxycillin. However, with the advent of the twice-daily formulations of amoxycillin+clavulanate, these effects have been reduced because of the lower daily dose of clavulanic acid. See also p.21 and p.22.

For precautions and interactions, see p.21.

Cephalosporins

The cephalosporins are best categorised according to their antimicrobial activities rather than their 'generations'.

Cephalexin and **cephazolin** are moderate-spectrum cephalosporins without anti-*Haemophilus* activity. They are similar in their range of antimicrobial activity. They are active against streptococci and staphylococci, including beta-lactamase–producing staphylococci, but are inactive against enterococci and *Listeria monocytogenes*. Their Gram-negative spectrum includes most *Escherichia coli* and *Klebsiella* species, but they are inactive against many Gram-negative aerobes (eg *Serratia*, *Enterobacter* and *Pseudomonas* species). They are not useful against the Gram-negative anaerobe *Bacteroides fragilis* and related species.

For other cephalosporins and their categories, see Table 1 (p.16).

For precautions, see p.21.

Adverse effects: The major adverse effects of cephalosporins are hypersensitivity (allergy) (see p.15), resistance (see p.15), and diarrhoea (see p.17). The common adverse effects are diarrhoea, nausea, rash, eosinophilia, drug fever, electrolyte disturbances, and pain and inflammation (at the injection site).

Interactions: The most significant interaction of the cephalosporins is with warfarin, and therefore the patient's INR (international normalised ratio) should be monitored when parenteral cephalosporins are administered.

Nitroimidazoles

Metronidazole and **tinidazole** are nitroimidazoles. Nitroimidazoles have a spectrum of activity that encompasses Gram-negative anaerobes such as *Bacteroides fragilis*, Gram-positive anaerobes such as *Clostridium* species, and anaerobic protozoa including *Trichomonas vaginalis*, *Giardia lamblia* (*intestinalis*) and *Entamoeba histolytica*. Metronidazole is the drug of choice in spreading neck infection and acute ulcerative gingivitis.

Metronidazole is absorbed well, so tablets or suppositories can be used. It is also available as an intravenous preparation. Tinidazole, available only as an oral preparation, has a longer half-life than metronidazole and can therefore be administered as a single dose.

In these guidelines, for the treatment of mixed aerobic and anaerobic infection, metronidazole is recommended in a dose of 400 mg orally and 500 mg intravenously, with a 12-hourly dosing schedule. This is based on pharmacokinetic data and minimum inhibitory concentrations of the pathogens involved, to increase adherence (compliance).

Adverse effects: The most common adverse effects of the nitroimidazoles are nausea, diarrhoea, and a metallic taste.

Interactions: Nitroimidazoles can interact with alcohol causing a disulfiram-like reaction (severe intestinal cramping, sweating, nausea and vomiting) and patients must be counselled to avoid alcohol during the course of treatment. Metronidazole also enhances the activity of warfarin, and the patient's INR (international normalised ratio) should be monitored.

Glycopeptides

Vancomycin and **teicoplanin** are glycopeptides. Glycopeptides are active against a wide range of Gram-positive organisms; Gram-negative organisms are not susceptible. Glycopeptides are sometimes used to treat severe infection with susceptible organisms in patients hypersensitive to penicillin. Vancomycin may be used for prophylaxis of endocarditis in patients hypersensitive to penicillins.

Adverse effects: The most common adverse effects of the glycopeptides are itch, fever, chills, eosinophilia, mild gastrointestinal tract disturbances (with oral vancomycin), pain, erythema, thrombophlebitis and nephrotoxicity.

Lincosamides

Clindamycin and **lincomycin** are lincosamides. Lincosamides are active against Gram-positive aerobes and most anaerobes. These drugs are used as second-line therapy. A parenteral formulation is available for lincomycin. Oral clindamycin is available, but there is no paediatric oral formulation currently marketed in Australia. Intravenous doses should be administered slowly to avoid producing serious arrhythmias.

Adverse effects: The most common adverse effects of the lincosamides are diarrhoea (see p.17), nausea, vomiting, abdominal cramps, abdominal pain, metallic taste (with intravenous administration), itch, rash and contact dermatitis (with topical administration).

Macrolides

Azithromycin, **clarithromycin**, **erythromycin** and **roxithromycin** have a wide spectrum of activity covering Gram-positive cocci, *Legionella*, *Bordetella* (not roxithromycin), *Corynebacteria*, Gram-negative cocci, *Mycoplasma*, *Chlamydia* and both Gram-positive and Gram-negative anaerobes, but not enteric Gram-negative rods.

The newer macrolides have more reliable absorption and longer half-lives (azithromycin > roxithromycin > clarithromycin > erythromycin), which allows less frequent dosing. The newer macrolides attain high intracellular concentrations that confer theoretical benefits in the treatment of infections caused by intracellular pathogens. Roxithromycin is preferred to erythromycin because it has a more benign adverse effect profile and fewer drug interactions. Roxithromycin is not listed in the dental section of the Schedule of Pharmaceutical Benefits; however, on a private prescription, it is not expensive.

Macrolides are rarely indicated in dental practice.

Adverse effects: The oral formulations of erythromycin have variable absorption and frequent gastrointestinal adverse effects. The newer macrolides have fewer adverse effects than erythromycin. The most common adverse effects of the macrolides are nausea, vomiting, diarrhoea, abdominal pain, cramps, headache, dyspnoea, cough and candidal infections.

Interactions: Erythromycin and clarithromycin are potent inhibitors of the cytochrome P450 enzyme system (particularly CYP3A4), so significant drug interactions occur (eg with carbamazepine, warfarin). Macrolides can increase absorption of digoxin. Co-administration of colchicine and clarithromycin or erythromycin has been associated with increased risk of fatal bone marrow toxicity. Erythromycin and clarithromycin (with the other macrolides being associated in case reports) have the potential to prolong the QT interval, which will potentiate that effect if used with drugs that have a similar tendency (eg sotalol, tricyclic antidepressants).

Tetracyclines

Tetracyclines have a broad spectrum of activity, which includes Gram-positive and Gram-negative bacteria, *Chlamydia*, *Rickettsia*, *Mycoplasma*, spirochaetes, some nontuberculous mycobacteria and some protozoa. They are usually bacteriostatic. Tetracyclines are contraindicated in children younger than eight years of age; however, because dentine development may continue beyond this age, some practitioners avoid use of tetracyclines in children up to the age of 12 years. Tetracyclines are safe for use during the first 18 weeks of pregnancy (16 weeks postconception) after which they may affect the formation of the baby's teeth and cause discolouration. Tetracyclines may be used for short courses (eg 7 to 10 days) in breastfeeding women if there are no appropriate alternatives.

Doxycycline is the preferred tetracycline in most situations, as once-daily dosing enhances adherence (compliance). Additionally, on a number of parameters, with the exception of possible photosensitivity, it is the least toxic of all the tetracyclines.

Precautions: Oesophagitis can occur with doxycycline, so it should be washed down with a glass of water and the patient should be instructed to remain upright for at least 30 minutes after oral administration.

Warnings: Patients should be advised of possible photosensitivity, and sun protection should be recommended.

Adverse effects: The most common adverse effects of tetracyclines are nausea, vomiting, epigastric burning, skin pigmentation, and tooth discolouration, bone deformity and reduced bone growth in children younger than eight years. Candidal overgrowth can occur with any tetracycline. Photosensitivity reactions can occur with any tetracyclines, but are most likely with doxycycline. Oesophagitis can occur with any tetracycline.

Interactions: There are several important interactions with tetracyclines. Antacids decrease absorption of tetracyclines, and oral doses of tetracyclines and antacids should be separated by two hours. Some drugs (eg carbamazepine, phenytoin) reduce plasma levels of doxycycline. Urinary alkalisers increase renal elimination of tetracyclines. Tetracyclines enhance the activity of warfarin, and the patient's INR (international normalised ratio) should be monitored.

Antifungal drugs

Azoles

Bifonazole, **clotrimazole**, **econazole**, **ketoconazole** and **miconazole** are used in the treatment of mucocutaneous candidosis, dermatophytosis and pityriasis versicolor. Clotrimazole has some activity against trichomonas, and ketoconazole shampoo is used in the treatment of seborrhoeic dermatitis and dandruff.

Ketoconazole, **fluconazole**, **itraconazole** and **voriconazole** are used systemically for fungal infections. Ketoconazole is active against a variety of fungal infections, particularly yeasts. Fluconazole has activity against *Cryptococcus*. Itraconazole has a broader spectrum, being active also against *Aspergillus* species. Voriconazole is active against *Aspergillus* species, *Scedosporium apiospermum* and *Fusarium* species. Miconazole is occasionally used intravenously in the treatment of rare systemic fungal infections.

Fluconazole has good tissue penetration, including penetration into the central nervous system. It is well absorbed following oral administration, but is expensive.

Itraconazole absorption requires an acidic stomach pH. Absorption is decreased in patients on proton pump inhibitors or histamine$_2$-receptor antagonists and an alternative antifungal is more appropriate in these patients. The oral capsule formulation achieves high levels if taken with a full meal; however, the oral solution is best absorbed on an empty stomach.

Ketoconazole has similar acid-dependent oral absorption to itraconazole and is not significantly excreted in the urine.

Miconazole is available as a topical 2% oral gel, which is used to treat oral candidosis.

Patients using topical antifungal agents should be counselled to continue treatment for seven days after symptoms have disappeared, to prevent the germination of the remaining spores that invariably are present.

Adverse effects: Adverse effects of the azoles include hepatotoxicity and hypoadrenalism. Liver function needs to be monitored monthly in patients taking systemic azoles.

Interactions: Systemic ketoconazole, itraconazole, fluconazole and voriconazole inhibit the metabolism of drugs metabolised by several cytochrome P450 enzymes (eg carbamazepine, warfarin), potentially increasing the effects of these drugs. Even topical applications of an azole (such as miconazole on the oral mucosa or gingiva) may cause a significant increase in INR (international normalised ratio) when used in patients taking warfarin.

Polyenes

Amphotericin and **nystatin** are polyene antifungal agents. Amphotericin can be used systemically for severe systemic fungal infections. Nystatin is rarely used systemically, because of its toxicity. Both are highly effective against *Candida* species.

In addition to their topical use on skin, amphotericin and nystatin can be used topically on oral mucosa, because they are not absorbed through mucosa or the gastrointestinal tract to any significant levels. They are available as tablets, lozenges and creams; nystatin is also available as oral drops.

Adverse effects: There are few adverse effects of oral polyenes. The most common are mild gastrointestinal symptoms (nausea, vomiting, diarrhoea).

Antiviral drugs

Guanine analogues

Aciclovir, **famciclovir**, and **valaciclovir** are active against herpes simplex and varicella-zoster virus. Aciclovir is absorbed poorly and erratically from the gut, and even less through the skin. Valaciclovir, a prodrug of aciclovir, has improved bioavailability compared with aciclovir. Famciclovir is is well absorbed from the gut.

Aciclovir is used topically, either alone or in combination with topical anaesthetics, for the treatment of cutaneous herpes simplex virus infection.

Thymidine analogues

Idoxuridine is used topically in the treatment of cutaneous herpes simplex virus infection. It should only be used in the prodromal phase and the first 48 hours of infection.

ANALGESICS

Three broad groups of drugs are used as analgesics for dental and oral pain—anti-inflammatory drugs, paracetamol, and opioids (also known as narcotics).

Anti-inflammatory drugs are very useful adjuncts to dental treatment because they provide therapeutic action at the site of the inflammation. Anti-inflammatory drugs can be classified into two groups—nonsteroidal anti-inflammatory drugs (NSAIDs) and corticosteroids. The choice of drug depends on the action required, although a corticosteroid is rarely required for inflammation of dental origin.

Nonsteroidal anti-inflammatory drugs

General considerations

Drugs belonging to the nonsteroidal anti-inflammatory drug (NSAID) group are the most commonly used drugs for pain relief. Many patients use NSAIDs for self-management of common pain problems (eg headaches, muscular aches, period pain, toothache).

NSAIDs are effective for the relief of nociceptive pain associated with tissue damage and inflammation. The traditional belief is that the main effect of these drugs is to inhibit cyclo-oxygenase (COX), which in turn reduces the synthesis of pro-inflammatory mediators (prostaglandins) from arachidonic acid. However, recent work suggests that there may be additional mechanisms of action. NSAIDs act both at peripheral sites in the body (ie where the tissue damage has occurred) and in the central nervous system. Evidence exists to indicate that an NSAID should be the drug of first choice for acute dental pain.

The dose of NSAID used affects its performance, particularly its anti-inflammatory action. Lower doses can provide pain relief, but higher doses are required for effective anti-inflammatory action (eg a single dose of 200 mg ibuprofen may relieve pain temporarily, but at least 400 mg is required to reduce the inflammatory response; it is even more effective with 600 mg or 800 mg). The time interval of the drug doses is important to maintain blood levels at a level that reduces the inflammatory response. These drugs should be used as a 'course of treatment' with regular doses at the correct time intervals rather than just when the patient feels pain or discomfort. It is important to educate the patient about how to use these drugs properly.

Ibuprofen produces greater analgesia than paracetamol+codeine combinations, and produces a dose-related analgesia over the range of 200 mg to 800 mg (ie increasing the dose from 400 mg to 600 mg will provide better pain relief, as will increasing it from 600 mg to 800 mg). However, adverse effects are also dose-related, and therefore the analgesic needs of the patient must be balanced with the risk of producing adverse effects.

NSAIDs are indicated for mild to moderate pain and are particularly effective for bone pain, which makes them very useful for many dental conditions. However, severe pain usually requires the additional use of another analgesic, such as paracetamol.

Adverse effects: Information regarding toxicity associated with NSAIDs is evolving, and remains somewhat unclear. All NSAIDs have potential adverse effects; these are shown in Table 2. The potential adverse effects should be discussed with the patient. In patients who require NSAIDs, particularly where risk factors are present, strategies may be needed to reduce the risk of gastrointestinal toxicity (risk factors for developing NSAID-associated gastrointestinal toxicity are listed in Box 5, p.32). Aspirin is contraindicated in children because it has been implicated as a cause of Reye's syndrome (a disorder of hepatic and central nervous system function).

Interactions: NSAIDs interact with many drugs, including angiotensin converting enzyme (ACE) inhibitors, angiotensin II receptor antagonists, inhibitors of some cytochrome P450 enzymes, some diuretics, lithium and warfarin.

Precautions: NSAIDs are available both as over-the-counter medications and on prescription; they are packaged in different dosages for different markets. It is important that the prescriber prescribes the correct dosage *and* explains the potential problems to the patient. Some commercial formulations combine NSAIDs with other drugs; hence a careful history needs to be taken to determine a total daily dose of each component. See also 'Adverse effects' (above) and 'Risk factors for developing NSAID-associated gastrointestinal adverse reactions' (Box 5, p.32).

Individual nonsteroidal anti-inflammatory drugs

There are many different NSAIDs available. They have similar efficacy; hence, the choice of which drug to use is largely based on safety,

Table 2. Adverse effects of nonsteroidal anti-inflammatory drugs

System	Adverse effects
cardiovascular	rise in blood pressure, fluid retention, myocardial infarction
neurological	headaches, confusion, hallucinations, depersonalisation reactions, depression, tremor, aseptic meningitis, tinnitus, vertigo, neuropathy, toxic amblyopia, transient transparent corneal deposits
gastrointestinal	nausea, vomiting, dyspepsia, diarrhoea, constipation, gastric mucosal irritation, superficial erosions, peptic ulceration, oesophagitis and strictures, faecal blood loss, major gastrointestinal haemorrhage, penetrating ulcers, small bowel erosions (see also Box 5, p.32)
haematological	anaemia, bone marrow depression, decreased platelet aggregation
hepatic	hepatotoxicity, fulminant hepatic failure
renal	glomerulopathy, interstitial nephritis, changes in renal blood flow leading to a fall in glomerular filtration rate, alterations in tubular function, reduction in diuretic-induced natriuresis, inhibition of renin release, oedema
other	precipitation of asthma in patients with nasal polyps, skin rashes

availability, cost, and the route of administration required. The most commonly used NSAIDs for dental, oral and facial pain are ibuprofen and aspirin.

The pharmacokinetics of the NSAIDs vary considerably and details can be obtained from appropriate publications. Important data for the most commonly used NSAIDs in dentistry are given below.

Aspirin

Aspirin has a dose range of 300 to 900 mg, every 4 to 6 hours up to a daily maximum of 3600 mg. The time to peak blood levels is 1 to 2 hours; its elimination half-life is 0.25 hours but increases with dose (so as the daily dose reaches 2 g and above, the dosing interval can be increased). Aspirin is contraindicated in children because it has been implicated as a cause of Reye's syndrome (a disorder of hepatic and central nervous system function).

For adverse effects, interactions and precautions, see p.30.

> **Box 5. Risk factors for developing NSAID-associated gastrointestinal adverse reactions***
>
> Concomitant use of multiple NSAIDs
>
> Concomitant use of anticoagulants
>
> Age over 65 years
>
> Irregularity of feeding, or not taken with food
>
> Treated heart failure
>
> Treated diabetes
>
> History of peptic ulcer
>
> High NSAID dose (more than 120% of average daily dose)
>
> History of gastrointestinal bleed
>
> Presence of an alcohol-related illness
>
> Concomitant use of corticosteroids
>
> History of prior use of H_2-receptor antagonist
>
> Regular use of aspirin and other NSAIDs
>
> Cigarette smoking
>
> * in decreasing order of importance

Ibuprofen

If ibuprofen is required following dental treatment, a dose range of 200 to 600 mg every 4 to 6 hours up to a daily maximum of 2400 mg can be used for a short time (up to 24 hours). A higher dose (600 to 800 mg) can be used as a loading dose for severe pain. The time to peak blood levels is 0.5 to 1.5 hours; its elimination half-life is 2 to 2.5 hours. The dose range of ibuprofen for children is 5 to 10 mg/kg every 6 to 8 hours (to a maximum daily dose of 2400 mg).

For adverse effects, interactions and precautions, see p.30.

Naproxen

The dose range for naproxen is 250 to 500 mg, every 12 hours up to a daily maximum of 1250 mg. The time to peak blood levels is 1 to 2 hours; its elimination half-life is 15 hours. It is available both as an oral preparation and as a suppository.

For adverse effects, interactions and precautions, see p.30.

Paracetamol

Paracetamol is an effective analgesic drug that acts within the central nervous system. It also has some antipyretic action, but has no anti-inflammatory effects because it does not inhibit prostaglandins to any extent in the peripheral tissues when used at normal therapeutic doses.

Indications for paracetamol include:
- mild pain, particularly of soft tissue and musculoskeletal origin
- mild to moderate post-treatment pain
- severe pain, to supplement the use of opioids, allowing a possible reduction in opioid dosage
- fever
- an alternative to aspirin (eg when aspirin is contraindicated—hypersensitivity, hyperuricaemia, gastrointestinal bleeding or ulceration).

Paracetamol is rapidly absorbed and peak blood levels are reached within 0.5 to 1.5 hours; its elimination half-life is 2 to 3 hours. It readily crosses into the cerebrospinal fluid and to the brain where it has its major analgesic effect.

The typical dose schedule for healthy adult patients is 0.5 to 1 g every 4 to 6 hours up to 4 g per day (less in the elderly and the frail). Some oral preparations are modified for slow release, and can be taken every 8 hours.

Formulations include standard tablets and capsules, an extended-action formulation, chewable tablets, soluble and effervescent tablets, oral solution and suspensions, suppositories, and an injectable formulation. Soluble, sustained-release and suppository formulations of paracetamol are all more expensive per unit dose than the standard tablet or capsule. Clinicians should be familiar with the range of over-the-counter preparations so they can accurately advise patients.

Precautions: Paracetamol is metabolised in the liver (the metabolites are excreted by the kidneys), and so its use in patients with liver disease should be restricted. Paracetamol is available as various formulations and under many brand names both alone and as combination preparations. It is also an ingredient in many nonprescription medications (eg cold and flu preparations). Inadvertent overdose due to ingestion of higher than recommended doses is a possibility, and patients should be advised to consider the paracetamol content of all medications being taken; a careful history needs to be taken to determine a total daily dose of paracetamol.

Adverse effects and interactions: Paracetamol is generally considered a safe analgesic with few adverse effects compared with other drugs. There may be an increased risk of upper gastrointestinal complications with paracetamol doses greater than 2 g daily (especially when used in conjunction with NSAIDs), and an increased risk of hypertension in women. Care needs to be taken in patients taking anticoagulants. Rarely, patients may experience urticarial or erythematous rashes, fever or blood dyscrasias.

Overdose: With high doses (single doses of more than 100 mg/kg), paracetamol can produce severe hepatotoxicity, hypoglycaemia and acute renal tubular necrosis. In adults, a dose of about 7.5 to 15 g (fifteen to thirty 0.5 g tablets), ingested and fully absorbed, is considered potentially toxic. Much lower doses may be toxic in patients suffering from starvation, fasting or other acute hepatic insult. The smallest fatal dose recorded in adults is 18 g. A paracetamol overdose is a medical emergency that requires recognition and prompt management. Clinical signs of the severity of the overdose may take some days to develop, so hepatic and renal function tests and plasma paracetamol concentration should be performed immediately and be monitored.

Opioids (narcotics)

Opioids are generally used for severe pain (eg severe postoperative pain, severe acute trauma, chronic cancer-related pain). Opioids include codeine (the most commonly prescribed opioid in dental practice), pethidine, morphine, fentanyl, oxycodone, methadone and tramadol. Opioids have many significant adverse effects in all major systems of the body (see Table 3), and therefore should be used with caution.

Opioids act on specific receptors in the central nervous system, and can block all forms of pain, not just pain arising from tissue damage and inflammatory processes. The normal clinical doses used also dampen the patient's emotional response to the pain, perhaps more effectively than blocking the pain itself (ie the pain may still be noted by the patient but they are able to tolerate it or cope with it better).

Adverse effects: The adverse effects of opioids are summarised in Table 3. Hypersensitivity may manifest as pruritus, urticaria, rash or bronchospasm. Opioid withdrawal syndrome includes body aches, diarrhoea, 'goose flesh', loss of appetite, nervousness or restlessness, runny nose, sneezing, tremors or shivering, stomach cramps, nausea, sleeplessness, diaphoresis, yawning, asthenia, tachycardia and unexplained fever.

Table 3. Adverse effects of opioids

System	Adverse effects
respiratory	dose-related respiratory depression (which is more marked during sleep or with concomitant sedatives, hypnotics, alcohol and general anaesthetics)
	bronchospasm due to histamine release
cardiovascular	bradycardia due to stimulation of the vagal nucleus in the medulla
	histamine release by morphine, morphine analogues and pethidine, which may cause vasodilation and hypotension during intravenous administration
	postural hypotension from peripheral vasodilation and baroreflex inhibition
neurological	dose-dependent mental clouding, delirium, sedation, nausea and vomiting, cough suppression, miosis, respiratory depression or apnoea, excitatory phenomena with myoclonus with high doses relative to renal function, reactivation of herpes simplex (with spinal and epidural morphine)
	following intraspinal use of morphine or hydromorphone, central adverse effects may be considerably delayed (6 to 12 hours)
dermatological	sweating, flushing
	urticaria and pruritus due to histamine release
gastrointestinal	vomiting, anorexia, decreased gastric motility, increased antral tone, delayed gastric emptying, biliary colic due to spasm of sphincter of Oddi and raised intrabiliary pressure, slowed digestion, prolonged intestinal transit time, increased anal sphincter tone, constipation; these are caused by mu- and delta-receptor agonists acting locally and centrally
musculoskeletal	chest wall rigidity (with fentanyl and fentanyl analogues), myoclonus
neuroendocrine	hypothalamic effects (including inhibition of gonadotrophin-releasing hormone and corticotrophin-releasing factor) leading to decreased gonadotrophins, adrenocorticotrophic hormone, beta-endorphin, testosterone, and cortisol; and increased prolactin
	antidiuretic hormone release is variably increased or inhibited by mu- and kappa-receptor agonists respectively
urinary	urinary retention and difficulty with micturition, increased external sphincter tone, decreased detrusor muscle tone, antidiuretic effect (with mu-receptor agonists)

Interactions and precautions: Serious adverse reactions such as serotonin syndrome may occur if fentanyl, pethidine or tramadol is administered to patients receiving monoamine oxidase inhibitors (MAOIs). Other opioids should be carefully titrated in patients receiving MAOI therapy due to occasional unconfirmed reports of interactions. Concomitant use of central nervous system depressant drugs (eg sedatives, hypnotics, phenothiazines, anaesthetics and alcohol) may increase the sedative and respiratory depressant effects of opioids. Concomitant use of drugs with anticholinergic activity (eg tricyclic antidepressants, atropine) may increase the risk of severe constipation and/or urinary retention. Optimal analgesia is difficult to achieve in an opioid-dependent person, and specialist advice may be needed.

Codeine

Codeine is metabolised to morphine, which is responsible for most of codeine's analgesic action. Approximately 10% of Caucasians are poor metabolisers of codeine, and have no detectable analgesic effect from codeine. Codeine is available for oral, subcutaneous and intramuscular use, with 8 mg of oral codeine providing equivalent analgesia to 1 mg oral morphine. Codeine has an elimination half-life of 3 to 4 hours, and duration of action of 4 to 6 hours.

For adverse effects, interactions and precautions, see p.35 and above.

Morphine

Morphine is well absorbed orally. The elimination half-life of standard formulations is 2 to 3 hours, and the duration of analgesic effect is 3 to 6 hours. The metabolites are excreted renally, and so may accumulate in patients with renal impairment. Tolerance may develop rapidly, particularly in intravenous drug users in the absence of pain. Opioids other than codeine are not recommended in dental practice other than in the hospital setting.

For adverse effects, interactions and precautions, see p.35 and above.

CORTICOSTEROIDS

Corticosteroids are useful drugs for the management of many dental and oral inflammatory conditions. Their use must be based on a complete medical and medication history plus an accurate diagnosis of the dental or oral condition, as they should not be used when an infection is present or is likely to occur. Corticosteroids can be used intradentally (within a tooth), topically or systemically. The most effective route of administration should be chosen; this usually means using a locally delivered form of the drug rather than a systemically delivered form wherever possible. Thus, intradental or topical corticosteroids are preferred as they place the drug at the site of required action, which results in more rapid onset of action and less chance of systemic effects.

Intradental corticosteroids

Corticosteroids have been combined with antibiotics for intradental application in the management of pulp and periapical diseases. The corticosteroid component is included as almost all pulp and periapical diseases are inflammatory in nature. The antibiotic is used as these diseases are usually caused by the presence of bacteria within the tooth, pulp or root canal system.

There are two forms of corticosteroid-antibiotic compounds that are commercially available and that can be used intradentally—a water-soluble paste, and a hard-setting cement.

The choice of which form to use depends on the condition being treated and where the material is to be placed.

The corticosteroid-antibiotic **pastes** are used as an intracanal medication (within the root canal system of a tooth) during endodontic treatment. The paste can be used as an initial medication for rapid and reliable relief of pain when treating irreversible pulpitis. It is also used as an intracanal medication to reduce the periapical inflammation (acute or chronic apical periodontitis)—and hence the pain—that is often associated with irreversible pulpitis and always associated with an infected root canal system. The pastes are also used as intracanal medication in the prevention and management of several forms of root resorption (eg internal inflammatory resorption, external apical inflammatory resorption, external lateral inflammatory resorption). An additional effect of the intracanal use of corticosteroids is a reduction in the amount of external replacement resorption that occurs following tooth avulsion and intrusive luxation injuries, as corticosteroids inhibit the action of clastic cells.

The **cement** form of corticosteroid-antibiotic mixtures is used within the crown of a tooth as part of a cavity lining or base, as an indirect pulp cap, as a direct pulp cap, or as a pulpotomy agent prior to restoration of cavities in teeth that have reversible pulpitis (ie reversible inflammation of the pulp). Commercial preparations typically also contain various other substances (eg calcium hydroxide, zinc oxide, eugenol). The cement is presented as a powder and liquid which are mixed to form a paste that is placed on the dentine or exposed pulp; it then sets to form the hard cement.

Topical corticosteroids

Topical corticosteroids have anti-inflammatory and immunosuppressant effects that are useful in a number of skin and mucosal disorders. Modification of the naturally occurring hydrocortisone molecule has produced a large number of drugs with varying anti-inflammatory potency for topical and systemic use.

The potency of topical corticosteroids applied to the skin is assayed by the degree of vasoconstriction they produce when applied under an occlusive dressing. This depends on the concentration used, the intrinsic activity of the compound, and its ability to penetrate the barrier of the epidermis, which may be influenced by the vehicle in which it is applied. The assay permits topical corticosteroid preparations to be arranged in groups with similar potency. Such a ranking corresponds approximately with clinical effectiveness (see *Therapeutic Guidelines: Dermatology*).

The vasoconstriction assay is not directly translatable to the oral mucosa, but the principles are similar and it is a ready reminder of the potency of this group of frequently prescribed drugs. It is also a clear reminder of their potency when applied intraorally, and accordingly the care required. The mucosa in different sites has different permeability. Keratinised masticatory mucosa (on the palate, dorsum of tongue and gingiva) is less permeable than nonkeratinised lining mucosa (on the floor of mouth, and ventral surface of tongue). The cumulative effect of corticosteroids on the various areas depends on the frequency and duration of application.

Oral topical corticosteroids should not be used in the presence of infection without appropriate antimicrobial cover. Generally, any infection should be cleared before the use of a corticosteroid. Systemic contraindications include the possibility of tuberculosis. Caution is also required in patients with hypertension or diabetes.

The topical corticosteroids available for intraoral application and their uses are outlined in Table 4 (p.40). Creams are less effective in the mouth than ointments, and the ointment form is preferred. Clinicians should exercise caution with the entire range of corticosteroids and, generally, avoid potent agents unless very familiar with their use.

General principles of topical corticosteroid use

Corticosteroids have both anti-inflammatory and immunosuppressant effects and their use must be precise and controlled. When topical corticosteroids are used on the oral mucosa, systemic absorption is

> **Box 6. Points to consider when prescribing topical corticosteroids**
>
> Corticosteroids are best applied with the pad of a washed finger. Applicators, including cotton tips, are fibrous and in dealing with atrophic fragile mucosa may inadvertently damage the tissues.
>
> Apply to wet mucosa. Drying the tissues before application is a natural instinct, but tissue trauma must be balanced against any benefit of drying (which is minimal).
>
> A prolonged period of avoidance of food and drink seems logical, but unlike topical applications to the teeth, corticosteroid absorption is reasonably rapid.
>
> A convenient time for application is after mouth hygiene in the morning and at night.
>
> Patients readily become frustrated as the ointments will not adhere effectively. This is overcome by frugal application, brief gentle rubbing with the finger pad, and reassurance that this application to the area is all that is required.
>
> Patients using topical corticosteroids requiring special methods of application (eg sprays, adhesives) need additional explanations.

generally limited, and the systemic effects reported following the use of extensive occlusive dressings on the skin are rarely encountered. However, caution is required when potent topical preparations are used.

Most topical corticosteroids currently available in Australia are for external skin use and this is stated on the packaging. Patients must be made aware of the nature of the medication they have been prescribed and that the medication is safe for intraoral application when used as instructed. Patients also benefit from written confirmation of verbal instructions separate from the prescription, as the dispensing pharmacist may not be familiar with the oral use of these drugs and so may supply conflicting advice. (The drug may, on occasion, not be dispensed, on the basis that it is 'for external use only'.) Points that may be helpful in formulating a set of instructions for patients are shown in Box 6.

Topical corticosteroids can be useful at several stages in the management of mucosal lesions; however, they should not be used unless a clinical diagnosis has been made (and a diagnosis that requires the use of corticosteroids).

continued on p.42

Therapeutic Guidelines: **Oral and Dental**

Table 4. Properties of topical corticosteroids used on the oral mucosa

Drug	Strength	Form*	Clinical potency on oral mucosa†	Oral uses
hydrocortisone acetate	0.5%, 1%	ointment	mild	minor oral mucosal inflammation, cheilitis (not suitable for angular cheilitis)
triamcinolone acetonide	0.02%	ointment	moderate	oral inflammatory dermatoses
	0.1%	emollient dental paste in adhesive vehicle	moderate	inflammatory oral mucosal conditions (eg oral ulceration, lichen planus)
betamethasone valerate	0.02%, 0.05%	ointment	moderate	oral inflammatory dermatoses (eg aphthous ulceration, lichen planus) (use with caution)
	0.1%	ointment	potent	oral inflammatory dermatoses (eg aphthous ulceration, lichen planus) (use with caution)
betamethasone dipropionate	0.05%	ointment	potent	oral inflammatory dermatoses (eg aphthous ulceration, lichen planus, pemphigoid, pemphigus) (use with caution)

continued next page

Table 4. Properties of topical corticosteroids used on the oral mucosa (cont.)

Drug	Strength	Form*	Clinical potency on oral mucosa[†]	Oral uses
beclomethasone dipropionate	50 micrograms /application	aqueous suspension delivered by metered atomising pump	potent	if wide exposure required (eg erosive lichen planus, pemphigoid, pemphigus, desquamative gingival conditions)
methylprednisolone aceponate	0.1%	ointment	potent	oral inflammatory dermatoses (eg aphthous ulceration, lichen planus) (use with caution)
mometasone furoate	0.1%	ointment	potent	severe inflammatory mucosal conditions (eg erosive lichen planus) (use with caution)
combination corticosteroid and antimicrobial[‡]	per gram: triamcinolone acetonide 1 mg, neomycin 2.5 mg, gramicidin 0.25 mg, nystatin 100 000 units	ointment	moderate	mixed infections, inflammatory mucosal conditions with predisposition to candidosis (eg angular cheilitis)

* In the mouth, creams are *not* as effective as ointments.
† Potencies of corticosteroids when applied to oral mucosa are not the same as when they are applied to skin.
‡ These must not be used by patients with sensitivity to triamcinolone, neomycin, nystatin or gramicidin.

Getting to know your drugs

The patient must be given clear written instructions, be advised about potential adverse effects (see below) and be reviewed regularly. Caution must be taken with corticosteroid use in patients with certain conditions (see p.38), and they should be avoided if a viral disease is suspected. The treatment goals should be defined; these may be directed to:

- symptomatic relief only
- complete lesion resolution (eg for minor aphthous ulceration)
- resolution but with residual visible tissue changes (eg for major aphthous ulceration)
- clinical management of a chronic condition (eg for atrophic lichen planus).

Most mucosal lesions progress through several stages (eg an aphthous ulcer may be prodromal, preulcerative, ulcerative, or show signs of healing or advanced healing). The stage of the disease must be identified, as this will assist in determining the treatment. Consideration of the stage helps establish if a corticosteroid is indicated and, if so, the appropriate potency, the method of application, the frequency and duration of treatment, and the expected treatment outcome. Most mucosal disease conditions respond best to a topical corticosteroid when it is applied at the earliest phase (eg topical corticosteroids are most useful for aphthous ulcers when they are in the prodromal and preulcerative phases).

Adverse effects

Adverse effects of topical corticosteroids may be due to local effects on the skin or mucosa at the site of application or to systemic effects following absorption of the drug (see p.45 for systemic adverse effects). Potential local skin effects include:

- loss of dermal collagen, leading to skin atrophy, formation of striae, fragility and easy bruising
- telangiectasia (development of prominent blood vessels)
- promotion of infection
- idiosyncratic reactions (eg allergic contact dermatitis, perioral dermatitis)
- purpura (in the elderly).

The intensity of adverse effects increases with the potency of the preparation. Intraorally, adverse effects are somewhat hidden but they are noted readily on the face and the vermilion of the lips. Potent corticosteroids should *not* be used on these sites.

A number of oral mucosal diseases cause tissue atrophy, particularly on the tongue (eg lichen planus). Long-term use of corticosteroids on such sites compounds the disease-related atrophy. Caution is required to monitor patient use and compliance, and to regulate clinical use against the level of tissue and sensory morbidity experienced by the patient.

Penetration of corticosteroid to the dermis is greater on the face and where conditions mimic application under occlusion such as skin flexures and intertriginous areas. The use of the more potent corticosteroids on these sites therefore carries greater risk of local damage and they should be used with caution. Only mild corticosteroids (eg hydrocortisone) should be used on these sites. In certain circumstances, more potent corticosteroids (eg methylprednisolone aceponate) may be used intermittently on these sensitive areas for up to two weeks; however, the greater the potency the greater the risk of local adverse effects—particularly perioral dermatitis. If improvement does not occur after two weeks, do not persevere with treatment—reconsider the diagnosis and seek specialist advice.

With greater potency, there is also an increased risk of rebound on withdrawal.

Absorption of the more potent agents applied to large areas may cause suppression of the hypothalamic-pituitary axis and other complications usually associated with systemic corticosteroid administration (see p.45 for adverse effects of systemic corticosteroids).

The classification of potencies of topical corticosteroids is shown in Table 4, p.40).

The most common adverse reactions to intraoral topical corticosteroids are secondary candidosis, nausea, oral use not tolerated (eg because of unpleasant taste), refractory response, mucosal atrophy, delayed healing, and systemic absorption. Secondary candidosis occurs frequently in patients using topical corticosteroids orally; in most cases this can be anticipated, and preventive and interceptive strategies can be used concurrently. As a general principle, any adverse reaction may:
- interrupt treatment
- cause a co-morbidity
- distract the treatment goals from the primary condition to the adverse reaction
- distort the primary disease presentation.

An example where all of these occur is medication-related candidosis.

Systemic corticosteroids

Systemic corticosteroids are rarely indicated in dentistry. They are sometimes used in the management of acute inflammation; they are not very effective for chronic inflammation. Their use should be reserved for situations where no other anti-inflammatory medication has helped, and there are no contraindications to their use (including the patient taking a drug that might cause an interaction). The dental practitioner must consult the patient's medical practitioner and, possibly, refer to a dental specialist. Corticosteroids suppress the immune response, which may have adverse effects on the patient's health and wellbeing.

The metabolism of corticosteroids is enhanced by drugs that induce liver enzymes (eg phenytoin and carbamazepine). The metabolism of dexamethasone can be reduced by itraconazole.

Systemic corticosteroids should be used only when there are no signs of infection and no possibility of an infection developing. They may be useful in the management of severe postoperative swelling, severe trauma, periapical nerve sprouting and acute apical periodontitis following removal of an acutely inflamed pulp, and severe muscle inflammation associated with temporomandibular disorder. Occasionally they are used for mucosal lesions that cannot be managed with topical medications.

Wherever possible, the topical use of corticosteroids is preferred because the immunosuppressive effects are much less (see pp.38–43 for topical corticosteroids).

Dental and oral problems needing corticosteroids usually require only a short course of treatment (typically 3 to 5 days), particularly if the appropriate local dental treatment has been provided. If the problem has not improved within this time, the dental practitioner should review, and possibly revise, the diagnosis, and consider other treatment strategies. The dental practitioner should monitor the patient's progress while they are taking corticosteroids, because many oral and dental inflammatory conditions are the result of, or are associated with, an infection (bacterial, fungal or viral) that may rapidly exacerbate once the inflammatory and immune responses have been suppressed by the corticosteroids. Conditions not resolving within a few days may warrant referral for specialist assessment and management.

Oral **prednisolone** is well absorbed and undergoes significant first-pass metabolism in the liver. It is eliminated by liver metabolism and its plasma half-life is approximately 3 hours; however, the biological action is prolonged for up to 36 hours.

Prednisone is a prodrug of prednisolone; it is converted rapidly to prednisolone *in vivo* if liver function is normal. Prednisolone and prednisone are considered to be clinically equivalent and can be used interchangeably.

Dexamethasone is a potent corticosteroid that can be used for oral and dental inflammatory conditions in a low dose for a short time.

Systemic corticosteroids are rarely indicated in dentistry.

Adverse effects, interactions and precautions: The major limiting factor in the use of oral corticosteroids is the development of adverse effects, which may be extensive and are largely dose-related. Treatment with prednisolone or prednisone at doses greater than 5 to 10 mg per day for more than a few weeks may be sufficient to cause adrenal suppression. Common adverse effects occurring at doses greater than those required to cause adrenal suppression include metabolic effects (eg diabetes), gastrointestinal effects (eg peptic ulceration), osteoporosis, skin atrophy, risk of infection, and immunosuppression. A patient taking corticosteroids should have their corticosteroids increased before surgery. Addisonian (adrenal) crisis can present 6 to 12 hours after surgical stress in a patient taking corticosteroids who has not had them increased before the surgery.

LOCAL ANAESTHETICS (LOCAL ANALGESICS)

Two often-confused words are **analgesia** and **anaesthesia**. Analgesia is 'the removal of pain sensation' whereas anaesthesia is 'the loss of sensation in general' (including pain). This difference in meaning is often lost, with many people (and publications) using the terminology 'local anaesthesia' when 'local analgesia' is what is meant. Local analgesia is the effect that dental practitioners aim to achieve in normal clinical activity; however, 'local anaesthesia' is the term commonly used in medicine and dentistry, and is used in this publication.

General considerations

Local anaesthetics inhibit the generation of electrical impulses and their conduction along the neuronal axon membrane, by reversible blockade of sodium ion channels. There is a constant imbalance of sodium and potassium ions between the cytoplasm of neurones and the intercellular fluid. This is maintained at about 25 times more potassium intracellularly and 15 times more sodium extracellularly. This imbalance is maintained through the sodium pump protein in the cell membrane, which maintains the resting membrane potential of -60 to -90 mV.

Action potentials are promulgated along a neurone process through the rapid flux of ions against the resting gradient. This results in a positive spike in the membrane potential that is dependent on the sodium pump. Local anaesthetic drugs affect the movement of sodium ions across the membrane by blocking sodium channels. However, this blockade can only occur from the intracellular side of the channel and thus a local anaesthetic drug is required to move through the cell membrane of the neurone before being able to block action potential promulgation. The progression of local anaesthetic block relates to nerve fibre diameter, myelination and conduction velocity.

A local anaesthetic molecule comprises a lipophilic head, a hydrophilic tail and a linking intermediate chain. The intermediate chain may be:

- an ester (aminoester group) (eg procaine, amethocaine). Esters are metabolised predominantly by plasma pseudocholinesterase
- an amide (aminoamide group) (eg lignocaine, prilocaine, mepivacaine, bupivacaine). Amides are metabolised in the liver and should be used with caution in patients with significant hepatic impairment.

The properties of the two groups are summarised in Table 5.

Lignocaine, bupivacaine and mepivacaine have active metabolites, which may contribute to activity and to toxicity. Many metabolites are formed by the cytochrome P450 isoenzymes CYP3A4, CYP2C9 and CYP1A2. Doses of local anaesthetics may need to be reduced when they are co-administered with drugs known to inhibit these enzymes (eg azole antifungal drugs, some protease inhibitors, erythromycin, verapamil, fluvoxamine). Prilocaine is metabolised to ortho-toluidine (o-toluidine), which can oxidise haemoglobin to methaemoglobin. Prilocaine is best avoided in patients with methaemoglobinaemia.

Atypical plasma cholinesterase (pseudocholinesterase deficiency) is a hereditary condition (affecting 1:3000 people) that results in molecular differences in the pseudocholinesterases, resulting in the poor metabolism of the ester molecules and increasing the risk of adverse outcomes.

Table 5. Properties of local anaesthetic groups

	Ester group (eg procaine)	**Amide group** (eg lignocaine)
water-solubility	more water-soluble	less water-soluble
primary place of metabolism	plasma	liver
method of metabolism	by pseudocholinesterases	by de-ethylation

Adverse effects of local anaesthetics

Local anaesthesia is an effective and relatively safe method of pain control, and has a very low incidence of significant adverse effects. Different anaesthetic drugs can have different complications. The adverse effects of local anaesthetics include:

- central nervous system effects—light-headedness, nervousness, apprehension, euphoria, confusion, dizziness, drowsiness, blurred or double vision, twitching, tremors, convulsions and unconsciousness, difficulty swallowing, slurred speech, sensations of heat or cold
- respiratory effects—respiratory depression, respiratory arrest
- cardiovascular effects—bradycardia, hypotension, and cardiovascular collapse which may lead to cardiovascular arrest
- allergic responses—cutaneous lesions, urticaria, oedema, anaphylactoid reactions
- local complications (outlined on p.159)
- toxicity (see below).

There have been studies indicating that some components of different local anaesthetics have different incidence of complications. The summary above is a composite of the fundamental complications that can occur.

Toxicity

Clinicians using local anaesthetics should be familiar with the diagnosis and management of drug-related toxicity. Other acute emergencies can arise with nerve blocks. Resuscitation drugs and equipment, including oxygen, should always be available for the immediate management of adverse reactions (see p.188 for emergency drugs and equipment recommended for dental practitioners).

Systemic toxicity may arise after inadvertent intravascular injection of local anaesthetic, rapid systemic absorption, excessive dose administration or impaired drug clearance. Adverse systemic effects are usually seen in a continuum as plasma concentration increases. With the majority of local anaesthetics, minor central nervous system effects are seen before seizures or the onset of cardiovascular toxicity, and may act as a warning of serious events. Lignocaine can cause circumoral and tongue numbness, light-headedness, visual and auditory disturbances, generalised muscular twitching, loss of consciousness, tonic-clonic seizures, coma, respiratory arrest and cardiovascular collapse.

Longer-acting local anaesthetics, notably bupivacaine, can cause cardiovascular effects before any observed central nervous system effect. Changes in cardiac conduction, excitability, refractoriness, contractility and peripheral vascular resistance can occur at therapeutic blood concentrations. Higher concentrations lead to life-threatening atrioventricular block, ventricular arrhythmias and depressed cardiac contractility.

Major systemic complications

The recommended maximum doses are very important. It is very unlikely that an overdose will occur in adults. However, local anaesthetic overdose in children can occur relatively easily, particularly in younger children. Extra care is required to actually calculate the maximum dose for children. Signs and symptoms of overdose range from excitability, sweating, vomiting, nervousness, numbness, disorientation and loss of consciousness through to respiratory and/or cardiac depression.

Allergic reactions to aminoester local anaesthetics may be due to the drug itself, preservatives (eg methylparaben) or antioxidants (eg sodium metabisulfite), which are in some preparations. Allergy to the aminoamide local anaesthetics is very rare, but has been reported. Cross-sensitivity can also occur, as many foods, drugs and skin preparations contain similar preservatives. Positive skin testing to one local anaesthetic does not provide any information about other drugs.

Choosing a local anaesthetic

Efficacy for a particular drug is determined by its concentration at the site of action. This depends on dose and concentration injected, diffusion to the site if distant from the injection, and on removal by the circulation, which in turn depends on vascularity of the tissue. The latter can be modified by co-administration with a vasoconstrictor (eg adrenaline) (see p.49). Increased lipid solubility enhances absorption. Increased ionisation, which depends on the pKa of the drug and the pH at the site, decreases absorption. It is important to read the manufacturer's guidelines as the concentrations of the local anaesthetics and associated vasoconstrictors change as new products come on the market.

Figures for maximum safe dose are imprecise due to the influence of multiple factors. Use the lowest dose and concentration required to produce effective anaesthesia. Local anaesthetic solutions should be administered slowly.

The duration of action and maximum doses of the different local anaesthetic solutions are summarised in Table 6 (p.50).

Use of vasoconstrictors

The addition of a vasoconstrictor to a local anaesthetic solution allows a longer working time (by reducing the rate of loss of the anaesthetic solution to the general circulation) and a reduction of the dose necessary to achieve effective anaesthesia. It reduces the bleeding, which improves operator vision, and therefore quality of care. Local anaesthetics currently in use do not cause vasoconstriction, therefore a separate vasoconstrictor is commonly added. In current practice, adrenaline and felypressin are the vasoconstrictors most commonly used. Noradrenaline has previously been used; however, it has significant adverse effects, particularly increased blood pressure.

Local anaesthetic drugs

The duration of action and maximum doses of the different local anaesthetic solutions are summarised in Table 6 (p.50). There is wide variation in the maximum doses recommended in different publications. In addition, many guidelines have different maximum doses for local anaesthetics when used with and without vasoconstrictors. In this publication, the maximum doses have not been adjusted for the inclusion of a vasoconstrictor. Maximum doses are unlikely to be reached in most adult dental patients for most dental procedures, although this might not be so in children and the elderly.

Lignocaine

Lignocaine is an aminoamide local anaesthetic, and is also an antiarrhythmic drug. Lignocaine with adrenaline is the local anaesthetic most commonly used in dental practice. Allergy rarely occurs. See Table 6 (p.50) for duration of action and maximum doses.

Precautions: The dose may need to be reduced in people with impaired renal function or liver disease.

For adverse effects of local anaesthetics, see p.47 and p.159; for toxicity, see p.47.

Prilocaine

Prilocaine is an aminoamide local anaesthetic. It equipotent to lignocaine without adrenaline, but is less toxic and has a slightly longer duration of action. For dental use, prilocaine is often combined with the vasoconstrictor felypressin, which is contraindicated during pregnancy. See Table 6 (p.50) for duration of action and maximum doses.

continued on p. 52

Therapeutic Guidelines: **Oral and Dental**

Table 6. Duration of action and maximum doses of local anaesthetics used in dentistry

Drug	Duration (minutes)* pulp	Duration (minutes)* soft tissue	Maximum dose†	Approximate maximum number of 2.2 mL cartridges that can be used in a 70 kg person (and dose contained in it)
lignocaine 2% (20 mg/mL)	5–10	60–120	4.4 mg/kg to an absolute maximum of 300 mg in an adult	not available in cartridges in Australia
lignocaine 2% (20 mg/mL) with adrenaline 1:80 000 (12.5 micrograms/mL)	60–90	180–300	4.4 mg/kg to an absolute maximum of 300 mg in an adult	7 (308 mg)
lignocaine 2% (20 mg/mL) with adrenaline 1:100 000 (10 micrograms/mL)	60–90	180–300	4.4 mg/kg to an absolute maximum of 300 mg in an adult	7 (308 mg)
prilocaine 4% (40 mg/mL)	30–45	60–180	6 mg/kg to an absolute maximum of 400 mg in an adult	4.5 (396 mg)
prilocaine 3% (30 mg/mL) with adrenaline 1:300 000 (3.3 micrograms/mL)	30–90	120	6 mg/kg to an absolute maximum of 400 mg in an adult	6 (396 mg)
prilocaine 3% (30 mg/mL) with felypressin 0.03 international units/mL	40–90	150–210	6 mg/kg to an absolute maximum of 400 mg in an adult	6 (396 mg)

continued next page

Table 6. Duration of action and maximum doses of local anaesthetics used in dentistry (cont.)

Drug	Duration (minutes)* pulp	Duration (minutes)* soft tissue	Maximum dose†	Approximate maximum number of 2.2 mL cartridges that can be used in a 70 kg person (and dose contained in it)
articaine 4% (40 mg/mL) with adrenaline 1:100 000 (10 micrograms/mL)	60–75	180–360	7 mg/kg to an absolute maximum of 500 mg in an adult	5.5 (484 mg)
mepivacaine 3% (30 mg/mL)	20–40	120–180	4.4 mg/kg to an absolute maximum of 300 mg in an adult	4.5 (297 mg)
mepivacaine 2% (20 mg/mL) with adrenaline 1:100 000 (10 micrograms/mL)	60–90	90–180	4.4 mg/kg to an absolute maximum of 300 mg in an adult	7 (308 mg)
bupivacaine 0.5% (5 mg/mL) with adrenaline 1:200 000 (5 micrograms/mL)	90–180	240–540	1.3 mg/kg to an absolute maximum of 90 mg in an adult	8 (88 mg)

* variable, dependent upon dose and route of administration

† variable, dependent upon route of administration, medical history and many other factors. Maximum doses are unlikely to be reached in most adult dental patients for most dental procedures. This might not be so in children and the elderly. Maximum doses are expressed in terms of the local anaesthetic, not the vasoconstrictor. Many guidelines have different maximum doses for local anaesthetics with and without vasoconstrictors. In this publication, the maximum doses have not been adjusted for the inclusion of a vasoconstrictor (this is in line with the recommendations given in Malamed S. Handbook of local anesthesia. 5th ed. St Louis: Mosby; 2004). As with all medications, it is recommended that the clinician confirms details of dosages with the relevant data provided through the manufacturer

Adverse effects: Doses greater than 600 mg or 8 mg/kg can lead to reduced blood oxygen-carrying capacity and cyanosis, often with delayed onset. The main disadvantage of prilocaine is methaemoglobinaemia at high doses in susceptible patients. For further adverse effects, see p.47 and p.159; for toxicity, see p.47. Adverse effects can be extreme with respiratory or cardiac arrest.

Articaine

Articaine is an aminoamide local anaesthetic. It is usually mixed with a vasoconstrictor (commonly adrenaline). See Table 6 (p.50) for duration of action and maximum doses.

Adverse effects: For adverse effects of local anaesthetics, see p.47 and p.159; for toxicity, see p.47. Methaemoglobinaemia can occur with the use of high doses of articaine in susceptible patients. There may be an association between articaine and neurotoxicity.

Mepivacaine

Mepivacaine is an aminoamide local anaesthetic. It provides a relatively long working time. It has an extremely low incidence of allergy. See Table 6 (p.50) for duration of action and maximum doses.

For adverse effects of local anaesthetics, see p.47 and p.159; for toxicity, see p.47.

Bupivacaine

Bupivacaine is a long-acting local anaesthetic. It is used for infiltration, peripheral nerve and plexus blocks, and epidural and spinal anaesthesia or analgesia. Onset time is about five minutes after infiltration. See Table 6 (p.50) for duration of action and maximum doses.

For adverse effects of local anaesthetics, see p.47 and p.159; for toxicity, see p.47.

Vasoconstrictors

Information about the concentration of vasoconstrictors and the local anaesthetics they are used with is shown in Table 6 (p.50).

Adrenaline

Adrenaline used for dental procedures ranges in concentration between 1:80 000 and 1:300 000. It is a synthetic molecule with the same structure as endogenous adrenaline from the adrenal medulla. Synthetic adrenaline has the same effect as natural adrenaline (ie vasoconstriction of the skeletal muscle vessels, pupil dilation, bronchial dilation, skin vessel contraction).

Adrenaline is affected by heat and light. Consequently, cartridges should be stored as instructed by the manufacturers (which usually includes keeping them in a cool and dark place). It is recommended to use cartridges at room temperature. Some clinicians warm cartridges before use; if this is done, it is recommended that this occurs only immediately before use and not for a sustained period of time.

Interactions: Dental local anaesthetics containing adrenaline are best not used for patients taking monoamineoxidase inhibitors (MAOIs) as MAOIs and adrenaline can adversely interact.

Felypressin

Felypressin is a vasoconstrictor based on the pituitary hormone oxytocin. This is used in doses of approximately 0.03 international units/mL, and at these doses has minimal myocardial effects. Its lack of effect on the central nervous system makes it useful where adrenaline is contraindicated (which is rare).

Contraindications: Felypressin is contraindicated during pregnancy as its similarity in structure to oxytocin (the hormone responsible for labour) can result in some contraction of the uterus.

Adverse effects: At higher doses, felypressin may cause some coronary artery constriction.

SEDATIVE AND HYPNOTIC DRUGS

Depending on the dose administered, drugs classified as anxiolytics and sedative-hypnotics have the ability to calm a patient and relieve anxiety (anxiolytic effect), promote drowsiness (sedative effect), and induce sleep (hypnotic effect). Confusion in terminology and classification can be attributed more to marketing strategies based on pharmacokinetic profiles than to unique effects produced by these drugs. All sedatives and hypnotics are central nervous system depressants. Their effects are dose-related; as the dose is increased, patients experience anxiolysis, sedation and ultimately hypnosis. The most common sedative and hypnotic drugs used for oral sedation in dentistry are benzodiazepines and antihistamines.

Benzodiazepines

Benzodiazepines are the most commonly prescribed anxiolytic and sedative drugs because of their efficiency and their relatively low incidence of adverse effects.

Benzodiazepines are effective as both anxiolytics and sedatives. Their therapeutic effect is attributed to their ability to potentiate the inhibitory influences of the principal endogenous neurotransmitter, gamma-aminobutyric acid (GABA), in the brain.

There is little basis for the use of more than one benzodiazepine concurrently in any patient.

Benzodiazepines are generally rapidly and fully absorbed after oral ingestion with peak plasma concentrations occurring from 0.5 to 2 hours after administration. There are some differences in absorption rate between the various drugs.

Contraindications: Contraindications to the use of benzodiazepines include allergy, psychoses and acute angle glaucoma.

Precautions: Patients taking other central nervous system depressants (including alcohol) should be aware of the additive effects of benzodiazepines. Caution is necessary when prescribing benzodiazepines to patients with psychoses, neuromuscular disorders, or respiratory, liver or kidney disease. Benzodiazepines cross the placental barrier and are excreted in breast milk. The potential for developing tolerance, dependence, and withdrawal symptoms is an important consideration (see p.57).

Adverse effects: The main adverse effects of benzodiazepines are physical dependence (see p.57), precipitation of delirium, and memory impairment. They can impair performance and affect judgment, so driving and other skilled tasks can be impaired. They can cause dry mouth and blurred vision. After prolonged use, benzodiazepines should be withdrawn gradually. Older individuals are particularly vulnerable to the adverse effects of ataxia (with consequent falls and injury), confusion, memory loss and cognitive impairment. The most frequently reported adverse reactions following oral administration include transient drowsiness (especially in the elderly and the debilitated) and fatigue. Paradoxical reactions consisting of excitement, hallucinations and rage can occur, and are more likely in children and the elderly; they may be seen in teenagers.

Diazepam

Diazepam is a widely used sedative. It is also used as a muscle relaxant and in the treatment of epilepsy. It is available in tablets and in liquid form. Diazepam is reliably absorbed from the gut, with its effect becoming apparent after about 30 minutes. The optimum clinical effect is reached after one hour. A single oral dose of 10 mg for adults can be given one hour before the dental appointment. Diazepam's elimination half-life is prolonged, being 14 to 70 hours (with 30 to 200 metabolites); the primary metabolite, nordiazepam, retains significant central nervous system depressant activity.

Precautions: There is some evidence that the use of diazepam during the first trimester of pregnancy increases the risk of congenital malformations such as cleft palate.

Interactions: Diazepam is metabolised via the cytochrome P450 (CYP2C19 and CYP3A4) enzyme system, and may interact with drugs that inhibit these enzymes (eg ketoconazole). Omeprazole may have some effect on plasma levels of diazepam.

For adverse effects, contraindications, and further precautions, see p.54.

Temazepam

Temazepam has a relatively short elimination half-life (3 to 25 hours) and has no active metabolites.

For adverse effects, contraindications and precautions, see p.54.

Antihistamines

Histamine and many other inflammatory mediator compounds are released during type 1 (IgE-mediated) allergic reactions. Histamine released in this way stimulates H_1 receptors, which contributes to the signs and symptoms of this type of allergic reaction (eg redness, swelling, itching, sneezing, runny nose, nasal congestion, red eyes). Histamine H_1–receptor antagonists can be divided into two subgroups—sedating and less-sedating.

There are few real indications for the use of antihistamines in dentistry other than for sedation. Sometimes patients with 'toothache' may respond to treatment with an antihistamine if the pain is actually of sinus origin.

Of the many antihistamines available, those most commonly used in dentistry for sedation are **promethazine** and, less frequently, **trimeprazine**. Antihistamines are less effective than benzodiazepines as sedative drugs. The sedative effect of antihistamines is attributed to their action as antagonists at histaminergic and cholinergic receptor sites, countering the normal excitatory influences of the respective neurotransmitters within the central nervous system. Histamine and acetylcholine are among several neurotransmitters associated with neural pathways involved in nausea and vomiting. For this reason, antihistamines are useful antiemetic drugs.

Doxylamine is sometimes used to help in post-procedural pain management; its sedative action may help the patient cope with pain. It is available alone and in combination with other drugs (eg with paracetamol and codeine). It has a long half-life of 10 to 12 hours, and it should not be used as a drug of first choice for pain of dental origin.

Adverse effects: Many antihistamine drugs cause drowsiness. Patients must be warned that they may feel drowsy, and that they should not drive a car or operate machinery while taking antihistamines. Antihistamines also potentiate the effect of other central nervous system depressants (eg alcohol). The sedating antihistamines possess anticholinergic activity and can cause dry mouth, blurred vision, constipation and urinary retention. Their use can lead to a drying effect throughout the respiratory tract and a thickening of bronchial mucus. They should not be used where their anticholinergic activity is contraindicated (eg in patients with narrow angle glaucoma or prostatic hypertrophy).

Trimeprazine

Trimeprazine has been found to be particularly suitable for sedation in children. It has a reasonable antiemetic action. It is available in tablet and syrup form; the syrup is available in two concentrations. Trimeprazine frequently overcomes the fear found in younger children, which is often resistant to small doses of diazepam or temazepam. The duration of action of trimeprazine is 3 to 6 hours.

Contraindications: Trimeprazine should not be used where its anticholinergic activity is contraindicated (eg in patients with narrow angle glaucoma or prostatic hypertrophy).

Warnings: Patients receiving other central nervous system depressants, including alcohol, should be aware of the additive effects of trimeprazine.

For adverse effects, see above.

Promethazine

Promethazine has been used in the sedation of children, but its use as a sole agent in sedation is less satisfactory than that of trimeprazine. Promethazine is available as the hydrochloride in tablets, liquid, and injection. The duration of action of promethazine is 4 to 6 hours; it has an elimination half-life of approximately 8 hours.

Contraindications: Promethazine should not be used where its anticholinergic activity may be contraindicated (eg in patients with narrow angle glaucoma or prostatic hypertrophy).

Warnings: Patients receiving other central nervous system depressants, including alcohol, should be aware of the additive effects of promethazine.

For adverse effects, see p.56.

Dependence, tolerance and addiction

Drug dependence, tolerance and addiction can be of major concern to both patients and prescribers.

Physical **dependence** is an altered physiological state whereby repeated administration of the drug is necessary to prevent a characteristic withdrawal, discontinuation or abstinence syndrome. For some drug classes, withdrawal is not a risk factor for the development of dependence and addiction, while for others (eg benzodiazepines) continued use and dose escalation may result from the experience of withdrawal on cessation of use. Drug dependence is a behavioural syndrome in which individuals continue to take a drug in the absence of a therapeutic indication, often despite medical or social consequences, and they behave as if the effects of the drug are needed for continued wellbeing.

Tolerance is a physical state whereby, after repeated administration, a given dose of drug produces a decreased effect, or increasingly larger doses must be taken to obtain the effects observed with the original dose.

Addiction is a behavioural pattern of overwhelming involvement with the use of the drug and its procurement, and a high tendency to recidivism.

Patients with a current substance use disorder, particularly alcohol or opioid use, or a history of such a disorder, are at particular risk of developing benzodiazepine dependence.

If a drug use problem is identified, it is important to investigate the use of other substances, as multiple drug use is very common. A range of psychiatric disorders also occurs with greater frequency among patients with problem drug use. The most common are depression, anxiety disorders (particularly social phobias) and personality disorders.

See also p.11, for prescribing drugs of dependence.

MOUTHWASHES

A mouthwash may be recommended as:

- an antimicrobial to decrease the number of microorganisms in the oral cavity
- a topical anti-inflammatory agent
- a topical analgesic.

Mouthwashes may be used to decrease the severity of oral diseases such as periodontal disease, caries and mucosal disease.

The use of mouthwashes in periodontal disease is controversial. However, there are specific instances where a mouthwash can have a use (eg for short-term use in patients with gingivitis when inflammation restricts normal toothbrushing). It should be made clear to patients that the principal treatment for chronic periodontal disease is not the use of mouthwashes, but professional intervention with root planing of involved teeth and meticulous oral hygiene (see pp.97–101 for periodontal disease).

The use of mouthwash *alone* for oral hygiene is not recommended. Oral hygiene must be, principally, toothbrushing and dental flossing. Nevertheless, in patients at high risk for caries, there are significant benefits of the use of mouthwashes containing fluoride for prevention. These are discussed on p.93 and p.95.

The use of topical agents for oral mucosal disease is often the most effective treatment; this is discussed in 'Oral mucosal disease' (p.107) and in 'Topical corticosteroids' (p.38).

It had been recommended in the past that the use of an antimicrobial mouthwash pre-procedurally decreases the incidence of oral infections in patients, decreases the microbial content of aerosols present in the dental surgery during treatment thus reducing the incidence of cross-contamination between health care workers and patients, and decreases the number of microorganisms in dental-induced bacteraemia. In an extensive review of the literature that culminated in recommendations regarding infection control measures in the dental setting, the US Centers for Disease Control and Prevention found that there was no evidence to support the use of a pre-procedural mouthwash for any of the above reasons.

Use of alcohol in mouthwashes

An analysis of 27 topical medications currently available in Australia and recommended as anti-inflammatory and analgesic agents found that only six are alcohol-free (only one of which is a mouthwash). Many of the 27 products are recommended for children, and in most of the products, the level of alcohol is high (up to 40% w/v). In the most popular brands of mouthwash, the level of alcohol is 22% to 26% w/v. Alcohol causes profound drying of the oral mucosa, and thus patients with oral mucosal disease and xerostomia should avoid these products, as they will exacerbate their condition.

Epidemiologically, there is evidence to link the use of alcohol with the development of oral cancer. The association between alcohol-containing mouthwashes and oral cancer is far from established, with very few studies having sound methodology. A mid-1990s review of these studies concluded that there was no support for a link between mouthwash use and oral cancer. However, a more recent study[*] showed that the use of alcohol-containing mouthwash caused an elevated, but not statistically significant, risk for oral cancer among patients who neither smoked cigarettes nor drank alcohol.

Although the available data do not support a causative relation between mouthwash use and the development of oral cancer, there would appear to be no evidence to justify the use of alcohol in mouthwashes.

Individual agents

Mouthwashes containing fluoride are discussed on p.93 and p.95.

Chlorhexidine

Chlorhexidine is an antiseptic that is commonly used in mouthwashes. It is used as chlorhexidine gluconate in concentrations of 0.12% and 2%. It is also used in sprays, creams, gels, solutions, dressings and powders.

Adverse effects: Chlorhexidine salts can cause skin reactions, irritate mucosal surfaces, and interrupt wound healing. The mouthwash and oral gel can discolour teeth, margins of restorations, tongue and the buccal cavity; this extrinsic staining is not permanent and can be professionally removed. Chlorhexidine can also cause altered taste sensation, increased calculus formation, and mucosal irritation.

Povidone-iodine

Povidone-iodine is an iodine complex that has antibacterial, antifungal and antiviral properties. It is used in mouthwashes and gargles. It is also used in skin cleansers, and antiseptic creams, ointments, powders, solutions and paints, and in some antiseptic swabs and wound dressings.

---

[*] Winn DM, Diehl SR, Brown LM, Harty LC, Bravo-Otero E, Fraumeni JF et al. Mouthwash in the etiology of oral cancer in Puerto Rico. Cancer Causes Control 2001;12(5):419–29.

Adverse effects: Povidone-iodine can cause irritation of skin and mucous membranes. It is absorbed through damaged skin, therefore application over a large broken skin surface is not recommended.

Precautions: Povidone-iodine should not be used during pregnancy or lactation as it has the potential to cause hypothyroidism in the neonate.

Triclosan

Triclosan is a bisphenol antiseptic agent used in mouthwashes and toothpastes. It is also used in medicated soaps and topical preparations. It is a mild irritant, and allergic contact dermatitis has been reported.

Benzydamine

Benzydamine is an anti-inflammatory and analgesic agent structurally unrelated to the steroid group. It can be used for the temporary relief of painful inflamed oral mucosal conditions. It is available in mouthwashes, gels and sprays, sometimes in combination with chlorhexidine, in concentrations of 0.15% to 1%.

Adverse effects: Local adverse reactions of benzydamine, such as numbness and burning, have been occasionally reported. Systemic adverse reactions are very uncommon and are not serious.

FURTHER READING

eTG complete [CD-ROM]. Melbourne: Therapeutic Guidelines Limited [regularly updated].

Rossi S, editor. Australian medicines handbook. 2006. Adelaide: Australian Medicines Handbook Pty Ltd [regularly updated].

Tatro DS, editor. Drug interaction facts. St Louis: Facts and Comparisons [regularly updated].

Dental management of patients taking medications

Many patients presenting to a general dental practice are medically compromised and/or taking medications. These patients may have medical problems or be taking medications that can affect dental management. This section outlines some common and significant medical conditions, but only as they relate to patients fit enough to attend a general dental practitioner (ie the patient is not seriously ill, or hospitalised). The dental issues discussed with each medical condition are presented in a brief format for ready reference and are *not* a substitute for formal training or detailed texts. Medical emergencies may arise during dental treatment; these are presented in 'Medical emergencies' (p.165).

A detailed current medication list is an important part of the medical history (see p.2 for history-taking). If the patient is not sure what medications they are taking, they should be asked to bring in a list of their medications or obtain a current list from their medical practitioner or pharmacist. Crosscheck the medications with the medical history that the patient has provided, as there may be conditions that the patient has forgotten to mention or, as they feel well, they may have underestimated the severity of an underlying condition.

Before commencing dental treatment, careful consideration must be given to the appropriateness of this treatment to the patient's underlying medical problem. If the patient can tolerate only short periods of dental treatment, if their medical condition is easily destabilised or if their life expectancy is short, dental treatment should be modified appropriately.

CARDIOVASCULAR CONDITIONS

Cardiovascular diseases are common, particularly with increasing age. Approximately one-third of all Australians will die of cardiovascular disease. (See *Therapeutic Guidelines: Cardiovascular* for information on cardiovascular disease.)

Prevention of cardiovascular disease

Prevention of cardiovascular disease is aimed at the major modifiable risk factors for atherosclerosis (ie smoking, dyslipidaemia, hypertension, diabetes mellitus, sedentary lifestyle and obesity). The nonmodifiable risk factors are age, gender and family history.

The pharmacological methods of prevention include antiplatelet drugs (eg aspirin) and lipid lowering drugs (eg statins).

Dental issues

Dental practitioners should reinforce preventive strategies (eg smoking cessation).

The principal dental issues relating to cardiovascular disease are prevention of infective endocarditis (see p.135), and potential problems with anticoagulant and antiplatelet drugs (see below).

There are no dental drug interactions with statins (a lipid-lowering drug), but statins may occasionally result in an alteration of taste. This is an adverse reaction to the statin, but patients commonly think there is something wrong with their mouth.

Potential problems with anticoagulant and antiplatelet drugs

The key issue with patients taking an anticoagulant or antiplatelet drug is the balance between the increased risk of bleeding from a wound (if the drug is *not* stopped) and the risk of intravascular thrombi and emboli (if the drug *is* stopped). The emphasis in the past has been on minimising bleeding; however, the effect of an intravascular event is potentially much more serious to the patient. A stroke is a catastrophic event, whereas bleeding from the mouth, although messy and troublesome, can be easily managed by local means.

It is essential that the dental practitioner knows whether the patient is taking an anticoagulant or antiplatelet drug, which drug(s) they are taking and the current regimen, the underlying condition, and any other medications they are taking.

The most commonly used anticoagulant and antiplatelet drugs are aspirin and warfarin; others are heparin and clopidogrel.

For more information about dental treatment for patients taking an anticoagulant or antiplatelet drug, see the *Australian Dental Journal*[*] where this issue has been comprehensively reviewed.

---

[*] Carter G, Goss AN, Lloyd J, Tocchetti R. Current concepts of the management of dental extractions for patients taking warfarin. Aust Dent J 2003;48(2):89–96; quiz 138.

Aspirin

Patients taking aspirin have a normal INR (international normalised ratio) and a prolonged bleeding time.

Antiplatelet therapy with aspirin usually does not result in significant bleeding from extraction wounds. For dentoalveolar surgery (including extractions), there is no indication to alter a patient's regular aspirin dose. The risks and benefits of not changing the aspirin dosage should be discussed with the patient. Patients need to be warned that they may have a slightly higher chance of having some bruising but that this is a minor risk compared with the risk of embolic phenomena. Most patients prefer slightly increased bleeding rather than risk a cardiovascular accident or similar. It may be prudent to employ locally applied treatments (eg suturing, applications of local haemostatic agent) to help achieve haemostasis.

If aspirin *is* to be ceased, it should be stopped at least 10 days, and preferably 14 days, before the procedure, and restarted two days after the procedure. Stopping aspirin for only a few days or even up to a week before the procedure is of no benefit.

Warfarin

It is important that both the patient and their physician understand how the patient's warfarin treatment should be managed in relation to dental extraction. It is not uncommon for patients to reduce their warfarin dose without consultation or, alternatively, to consult with their physician who may (unnecessarily) wish to follow the traditional course of ceasing anticoagulants for minor surgery. See Box 7 (p.64) for procedures for patients taking warfarin who require minor oral surgery.

Hypertension

Risk factors for developing hypertension include age, hyperlipidaemia, cardiac events, diabetes and renal disease.

There are numerous medications available for the management of hypertension. Commonly these are used in combination.

Dental issues

Provided hypertension is controlled and stable, it usually is not a problem during dental treatment. Severe longstanding dental pain can increase hypertension, so appropriate dental treatment should be instituted promptly. Severe anxiety associated with dental phobia may increase blood pressure; in this circumstance sedatives should be considered. (See pp.161–4 for sedation.)

Box 7. Procedure for patients taking warfarin who require minor oral surgery

- Take a detailed medical history including:
  - dose regimen
  - stability of INR
  - underlying medical conditions
  - need for antibiotic prophylaxis.
- Organise blood test for INR within 24 hours before surgery:
  - If INR is less than 2.2 and there are no contraindications, proceed; tranexamic acid mouthwash is not required.
  - If INR is greater than 4.0, refer patient back to their general medical practitioner.
  - If INR is 2.2–4.0, proceed, using the tranexamic acid mouthwash protocol.

DO NOT CEASE WARFARIN.

Tranexamic acid mouthwash protocol (for patients with INR 2.2–4.0)

Day of surgery
- Obtain INR (INR must be 2.2–4.0).
- Administer antibiotic prophylaxis if indicated.
- Obtain bottle of tranexamic acid mouthwash.

During surgery (for extraction of teeth only)
- After teeth extracted, irrigate sockets with 4.8% tranexamic acid mouthwash* via a disposable syringe.
- Fill the socket with loosely packed haemostatic agent.
- Place one suture per socket.
- Get patient to bite on gauze pack soaked in tranexamic acid mouthwash.

After surgery
- Give patient tranexamic acid mouthwash with instructions on use (4.8% 10 mL for 2 minutes, 4 times daily for 2 to 5 days).
- Arrange review dental appointment for 2 days after the procedure.

Review appointment (2 days after the procedure)
- Note any bleeding, pain, delayed healing or infection, and deal with as necessary.

Review again 1 to 2 weeks later to ensure that there has been healing.

---

* If a 4.8% tranexamic acid mouthwash is not available, a 5% solution can be made by crushing a 500 mg tablet and dispersing it in 10 mL of water immediately before administration.

Theoretically, local anaesthetics containing adrenaline may elevate blood pressure; however, using a local anaesthetic without a vasoconstrictor, or using felypressin may be less effective for pain control than local anaesthetics with adrenaline, and thus may result in pain that may elevate blood pressure. Clinically, local anaesthesia with adrenaline gives good pain control with no clinically significant hypertensive effects.

Nonsteroidal anti-inflammatory drugs (NSAIDs) should be used with caution in patients taking antihypertensives, as there can be a risk of renal impairment. This risk can be increased if a patient is taking a combination of an angiotensin converting enzyme (ACE) inhibitor (eg enalapril) or angiotensin II receptor antagonist (eg candesartan) and a diuretic; the end result of the concurrent use of these three drug types may be renal failure.

Coronary ischaemic disease

Angina

The underlying problem that causes angina is chronic atherosclerotic obstruction of the coronary vessels, which is slowly progressive although the symptoms are often sudden. Severe obstructive coronary atherosclerosis restricts myocardial blood flow. When exercise or emotional stress creates a demand for more blood flow, this cannot be achieved because of the obstruction. Angina signals temporary myocardial ischaemia that subsides promptly with rest as the increased demand subsides.

Common medications used by patients that experience angina include glyceryl trinitrate (spray or tablets), antiplatelet therapies (eg aspirin) (see pp.62–3 for issues related to anticoagulant and antiplatelet therapy), and beta-blocker therapy (eg atenolol).

The management of severe angina is presented in 'Medical emergencies' (pp.167–8).

Myocardial infarction

Acute coronary syndromes (eg myocardial infarction) have the same underlying causes as angina, namely atherosclerosis. With a myocardial infarction, an atherosclerotic plaque abruptly becomes active with endothelial rupture, vasoconstriction, platelet adhesion, thrombosis and inflammation. The exact syndrome depends on the extent of thrombosis, distal platelet and thrombus embolisation, and resultant myocardial necrosis.

The management of acute myocardial infarction is presented in 'Medical emergencies' (pp.168–9).

Dental issues

The key issue with dental treatment for patients with a history of coronary ischaemic disease is to ensure that their current condition is stable and they are following their preventive and/or rehabilitation program.

Elective dental treatment should be deferred for three months after myocardial infarction, stent placement or coronary artery bypass surgery. If pain or infection occurs within the 3-month period following infarction, treat it as simply and expediently as possible. Antibiotic prophylaxis is indicated for extractions in the early phase, as there is still damaged endothelium present (see pp.135–43 for antibiotic prophylaxis).

The average length of effectiveness of coronary artery bypass surgery or cardiac revascularisation is 7.5 to 10 years. Thus a patient who has had a coronary bypass a decade or more ago may have returned to their pre–cardiac event state. If there is doubt, consultation with the patient's physician is appropriate.

Dental treatment should be modified to be effective but performed with minimum pain, stress and time. Use short appointments, relaxation techniques, and effective local anaesthesia with vasoconstrictors, and consider giving sedation (see pp.161–4 for oral sedation).

Epidemiological studies have implicated periodontal disease as a risk factor for the development of cardiovascular disease. Whether periodontal disease and cardiovascular disease are concurrent manifestations of vascular disease, or whether treatment of periodontal disease results in improved cardiovascular status remains unproven. The strength of the evidence is a current subject of debate with further studies needed. Regardless of the relation of periodontal disease to cardiovascular disease, improving dental and periodontal health is important.

Heart failure

Heart failure is usually a disease of the elderly. It can be predominantly left ventricular with pulmonary congestion and dyspnoea, or predominantly right ventricular with elevated venous pressure, peripheral oedema and hepatic congestion. Usually both coexist in the classical syndrome of congestive or biventricular heart failure.

Median survival following a diagnosis of heart failure is approximately 3 to 4 years. Only relatively recently has therapy been shown to affect survival—in particular the use of angiotensin converting enzyme (ACE) inhibitors, beta blockers and spironolactone.

Cardiomyopathy

Cardiomyopathies comprise a group of conditions where there is progressive failure of contractility of the heart muscle. They are managed with medications primarily to slow the rate and increase the strength of the heartbeat (eg digoxin) and with management of the associated cardiovascular sequelae. Cardiomyopathy is usually graded from stage 1 (being early and minor) to stage 4 (for which cardiac transplantation is the only treatment).

Dental issues

It is important for patients with heart failure that the condition is stable and the dental treatment is simplified to be appropriate for the medical condition. Dental procedures may need to be of shorter duration than for other patients. Patients with cardiac failure usually poorly tolerate being placed in the horizontal position, and should be kept with their head higher than their heart. A useful guide is to determine the extent to which the patient needs to be propped up in bed at night; if they can only comfortably sleep with the aid of multiple pillows, they may not tolerate the dental chair being placed horizontally.

Patients with advanced cardiomyopathy or heart failure may have valvular problems, and thus need to be considered for antibiotic prophylaxis for endocarditis (see pp.135–43 for antibiotic prophylaxis).

RESPIRATORY CONDITIONS

The most common and most significant respiratory disorder having an impact on dental management is asthma. Other important respiratory conditions are chronic obstructive pulmonary disease and obstructive sleep apnoea. (See *Therapeutic Guidelines: Respiratory* for general management of these and other respiratory conditions.)

Asthma

Asthma is a chronic inflammatory disorder of the airways which has an associated increase in airway hyper-responsiveness that leads to recurrent episodes of wheezing, breathlessness, chest tightness and coughing. The episodes are usually associated with widespread but variable airflow obstruction. Many of the symptoms of asthma overlap with other diseases (eg chronic obstructive pulmonary disease).

The prevalence of asthma is 12% in Australian adults and is higher in children. Asthma frequently presents in childhood, but can occur for the first time at any age. It is possibly underdiagnosed in older people.

The aims of medical management of asthma are to achieve good long-term asthma control. Medications that may be used include inhaled corticosteroids (eg fluticasone), short-acting beta$_2$ agonists (eg salbutamol), long-acting beta$_2$ agonists (eg salmeterol), oral prednis(ol)one, montelukast and sodium cromoglycate.

Acute exposure to specific substances (including drugs) in sensitised individuals can trigger attacks of asthma, and continued exposure can lead to persistent asthma. Common triggers are inhaled allergens, tobacco smoke, foods, food additives, and many drugs, as well as occupational factors.

Dental issues

The most important consideration in the dental treatment of patients with asthma is to avoid triggering an asthma attack during treatment. There are several drugs (eg aspirin and nonsteroidal anti-inflammatory drugs [NSAIDs]) that can cause bronchoconstriction in susceptible patients with asthma and they should be avoided or used cautiously. Paracetamol is the analgesic and antipyretic of first choice because adverse reactions are rare and tend to be milder than reactions to aspirin or NSAIDs.

Patients taking systemic corticosteroids require an increased dose of corticosteroid before their treatment if they have adrenal suppression (see p.74).

Patients may develop oral candidosis secondary to the use of inhaled corticosteroids. To reduce the risk of oral candidosis and systemic absorption of corticosteroids, patients who use inhaled corticosteroids should be advised to rinse their mouth and throat with water and spit out after inhalation. Patients using a metered dose inhaler (MDI) have the additional risk of dysphonia; these patients should be advised to use a spacer.

Patients who regularly use inhalers should be advised to bring them to dental appointments so that they can self-medicate if necessary.

If intravenous sedation or a general anaesthetic is required for a patient with asthma, it should be administered in a hospital by a specialist anaesthetist.

The management of acute asthma is discussed in 'Medical emergencies' (pp.171–3).

Chronic obstructive pulmonary disease

Chronic obstructive pulmonary disease (COPD) is characterised by airflow obstruction that is not fully reversible. The airflow limitation is usually progressive and associated with an abnormal inflammatory response of the lungs to noxious particles or gases, most commonly cigarette smoke. COPD usually has some combination of emphysema (where the lung parenchyma is structurally damaged) and airway damage (with airway wall thickening and narrowing of the airway).

Typically, COPD involves middle-aged or older people, and cigarette smoking is the major causative factor.

Dental issues

Dental treatment for patients with COPD needs to be modified depending on the patient's condition. Patients with COPD do not tolerate being placed in a horizontal position. Patients taking corticosteroids require their dose to be increased if there has been adrenal suppression (see p.74).

Smoking cessation is the only intervention that has been shown to improve the natural history of COPD; hence it is essential that the patient stops smoking. All health professionals should be actively involved in encouraging patients to stop smoking. Advice about smoking cessation is presented in *Therapeutic Guidelines: Cardiovascular* and on various websites (some available through the Australian Dental Association website <http://www.ada.org.au>).

Patients may develop oral candidosis secondary to the use of inhaled corticosteroids. To reduce the risk of oral candidosis and systemic absorption of corticosteroids, patients who use inhaled corticosteroids should be advised to rinse their mouth and throat with water and spit out after inhalation. Patients using a metered dose inhaler (MDI) have the additional risk of dysphonia; these patients should be advised to use a spacer.

Obstructive sleep apnoea

Obstructive sleep apnoea (OSA) affects approximately 4% of males and 2% of females. It is characterised by repetitive obstruction (apnoea) or partial obstruction (hypopnoea) of the pharyngeal airway during sleep. If OSA is not diagnosed and treated appropriately, it may lead to premature cardiovascular or accidental death. OSA has been reviewed in detail in the *Australian Dental Journal*.[*]

---

[*] *Sherring D, Vowles N, Antic R, Krishnan S, Goss AN. Obstructive sleep apnoea: a review of the orofacial implications. Aust Dent J 2001;46(3):154–65.*

Major factors in OSA are obesity and facial skeletal retrusion (eg retrognathia).

Treatment measures include weight reduction, smoking cessation, avoidance of night-time alcohol, avoidance of drugs causing sedation, treatment of nasal congestion, tonsillectomy, changing sleeping position, continuous positive airway pressure (CPAP), mandibular advancement splints, and surgery.

Dental issues

Dental practitioners have an important role in the multidisciplinary management of OSA, including the diagnosis of facial skeletal retrusion and the construction of mandibular advancement appliances.

Some patients with OSA can be effectively treated with a mandibular advancement splint; this must be performed in association with a multidisciplinary team led by a specialist respiratory physician.

Snoring can occur in isolation or can be a sign of OSA. It is not possible to diagnose whether a patient's snoring is due to OSA without a medical examination including sleep laboratory investigation.

> ***Using oral devices to treat snoring without such investigation is not appropriate.***

Patients with OSA are at particular risk of respiratory arrest under sedation or general anaesthesia, and any sedation or anaesthesia should be in a hospital with a specialist anaesthetist present.

ENDOCRINE CONDITIONS

Endocrine conditions of specific importance to dental treatment include diabetes, thyroid disorders, adrenal disorders, and osteoporosis when it is being treated with bisphosphonates. (See *Therapeutic Guidelines: Endocrinology* for general management of these conditions.)

Diabetes

Type 1 diabetes, which accounts for 10% of all diabetes, is primarily caused by immune-mediated destruction of the insulin-producing beta cells. Type 2 diabetes is multifactorial in origin, with risk factors including age, obesity, inactivity, pregnancy, ethnic origin and family history.

Typical symptoms of diabetes include polydipsia (chronic excessive thirst and fluid intake), polyuria (large amount of urine excretion), recurrent infection (including oral candidosis), and weight loss.

Patients with poorly controlled diabetes have an increased risk of periodontal disease and may have problems with oral candidosis, particularly related to the wearing of dentures. They should have regular dental care including instruction in oral hygiene measures and denture maintenance.

All patients with type 1 diabetes require therapy with insulin, whereas diet and regular exercise can often achieve good control of type 2 diabetes. If diet and exercise are not effective, therapy with one or more oral hypoglycaemic drugs (eg glibenclamide, metformin, rosiglitazone) may be prescribed.

Approximately 30% of patients with type 2 diabetes eventually require insulin; however, this is often not until after 10 to 15 years of successful use of oral medications.

Dental issues

Dentists should ascertain how the patient's condition is being managed by taking a thorough medical history.

Dentists should be aware of the possibility of undiagnosed diabetes in patients who show a sudden onset of periodontal disease or who show a delayed healing response to soft tissue treatment. Diabetes should also be considered in patients with recurrent or persistent bacterial or fungal infections. Provisional diagnosis is made by a fasting blood glucose test—organised by the dental practitioner or the patient's medical practitioner. Patients with an abnormal fasting blood glucose result should be referred to their medical practitioner for management.

Destabilisation of diabetic control

Most patients with diabetes have a routine of medications, diet, activity, and blood glucose monitoring that keeps them feeling well and their blood glucose within safe levels. Provided the routine is not interfered with, most general dental treatment can proceed uneventfully. However, some situations can cause instability (eg a prolonged sore mouth, such as occurs following dentoalveolar surgery, which can interfere with a patient's eating). This instability, particularly in a patient with unstable type 1 diabetes can cause a loss of diabetic control and the patient may require hospitalisation.

Patients with unstable type 1 diabetes require regular blood glucose monitoring and need alterations in their insulin dose. Patients often have their own blood glucose monitor and thus are aware of their current blood glucose levels. In this situation:

- it is reasonable to proceed with required dental management provided the patient with diabetes has a random blood glucose level (BGL) between 6 and 11 mmol/L (a normal random BGL range for a person without diabetes is 3 to 8 mmol/L)
- if the random BGL is above 12 mmol/L, the patient's diabetic medication needs to be adjusted by their medical practitioner
- a random BGL below 3 mmol/L indicates hypoglycaemia, and the patient requires glucose and should be treated by their medical practitioner as an emergency (see pp.177–8).

It is important to assess the patient's compliance with and understanding of the treatment of their diabetes. Essentially, the decision needs to be made before dental treatment as to what can be safely accomplished for a particular patient, or whether they require specialist treatment. Routine dental treatment for patients with stable diabetes is shown in Box 8.

Patients with type 1 or severe type 2 diabetes who require dental treatment under general anaesthesia need specialist medical supervision for preoperative fasting and their perioperative management.

Dental practitioners can inadvertently induce fasting by making the patient's mouth sore. Patients with diabetes must be advised that even if their mouth is sore, they must maintain their caloric intake, activity level and medication. They should be given advice on how to prepare food to a softer consistency if they are likely to have difficulty with eating.

The emergency management of hypoglycaemia is presented in 'Medical emergencies' (pp.177–8).

Problems with healing

In patients with undiagnosed, or severe and unstable diabetes, healing can be delayed and the risk of infection can be increased. Although there are no detailed studies showing clear benefit from antibiotic prophylaxis, consider antibiotic prophylaxis (see pp.140–1) for high-risk surgical treatments (see Table 14, p.137) in patients who require insulin. Antibiotic prophylaxis is *not* required for routine dental procedures.

Thyroid disorders

Hypothyroidism

Hypothyroidism is a common condition—particularly in females over 55 years, in whom the prevalence approaches 2%.

Hypothyroidism is generally managed with oral thyroxine.

> **Box 8. Routine dental treatment for a patient with stable diabetes**
>
> **Initial appointment**
> - Determine the patient's usual routine and what type of activity destabilises them.
> - Determine the extent and type of dental treatment required.
> - Ask the patient to bring their glucose monitor with them (if they use one).
>
> **Timing of treatment appointments**
> - Make treatment appointments for midmorning or early afternoon.
> - Remind the patient to maintain their usual meals and medications.
> - Avoid extensive treatments and prolonged appointments.
>
> **Treatment**
> - When the patient attends for treatment, check that they have followed their normal medication regimen. If they have missed a meal or scheduled snack, either have them make a different appointment time, or send them to eat, and treatment can be commenced 30 minutes later.
> - Do *not* give the patient glucose or a sweetened drink 'just in case'; this routine is usually ineffective and will disturb the patient's diabetes management for the rest of the day.
> - If the patient feels ill during treatment, cease treatment and assess the patient's blood glucose level with a blood glucose monitor (if available). (See Box 25, p.178, for the emergency management of hypoglycaemia.)
>
> **Do not allow the patient to leave your care if they are unwell or confused.**

Hyperthyroidism

Hyperthyroidism (thyrotoxicosis), has many presenting symptoms, ranging from the classical weight loss, heat intolerance, tremor, muscle weakness, and palpitations to more subtle atypical presentations, which occur particularly in the elderly. Treatment modalities of thyrotoxicosis include medications, radioactive iodine and surgery.

Dental issues

Patients with a stable medication-controlled thyroid disorder do not usually have difficulties with dental treatment. Despite statements in some older texts, there are no contraindications to the use of local anaesthetics with adrenaline as a vasoconstrictor.

Patients with an unstable thyroid disorder (particularly thyrotoxicosis) must have dental treatment deferred until their thyroid condition has been stabilised. Such patients, however, usually do not present in general dental practice and should be under specialist medical management. In patients with unstable thyrotoxicosis, local anaesthetics containing adrenaline are best avoided, as there is a risk of thyroid crisis.

Adrenal disorders

The adrenal glands produce steroid hormones from the cortex and catecholamines from the medulla. When the adrenal glands have been removed, or they do not produce sufficient amounts of cortical hormones (Addison's disease), replacement of steroid hormones, particularly the glucocorticoids, is essential. Catecholamine deficiency requires no replacement. Removal of one adrenal gland does not usually create the need for replacement of steroid hormones.

The most common cause of adrenal suppression is the medical use of corticosteroids, which are used in the management of some inflammatory and immune disorders (eg rheumatoid arthritis, severe dermatological conditions, severe asthma). Treatment with prednisolone or prednisone at doses greater than 5 to 10 mg per day for more than a few weeks can be sufficient to cause adrenal suppression.

There have been major changes in the prescribing of corticosteroids over the last two decades. In general, corticosteroids are much less frequently prescribed, and tend to be prescribed in short pulses rather than as a constant regimen. These changes have minimised the potentially profound adverse effects of corticosteroids and the problems associated with adrenal suppression.

Dental issues

It is important to know if a patient is taking corticosteroids, and what their underlying condition and current drug regimen are. If a patient requires constant high dosages of corticosteroids, there is generally a serious underlying condition. Consultation with the patient's treating physician is advised.

Dental treatment, particularly dental extractions, root planing and extended restorative treatment, may be physiologically stressful. If a patient with adrenal insufficiency cannot produce sufficient endogenous adrenocorticoids (particularly glucocorticoids) following such a stress, an adrenal crisis (Addisonian crisis) may occur. This presents as a progressive hypotension some hours after the stress. The patient may initially feel faint, then become confused and collapse. One way to monitor this situation is for the stressful dental treatment to be performed in the morning, and the patient remain for the rest of the day in the presence of a responsible adult who must be aware that if the symptoms occur they must contact the patient's medical practitioner. If treatment is performed in the afternoon, the condition may manifest at night and progress while the patient is asleep; this can result in death.

To avoid the complication of adrenal crisis, a patient with adrenal insufficiency should have their current dose of steroid increased on the day before and the day of treatment to simulate the normal increase in glucocorticoid secretion that occurs in response to stress. If a patient has been taking corticosteroids, the dose may need to be doubled. If the stress from treatment is more extensive (eg full dental clearance), or if accompanied by fasting or vomiting, the dose can be trebled or quadrupled.

The emergency management of adrenal crisis is presented in 'Medical emergencies' (Box 27, p.179).

Osteoporosis

Osteoporosis is common, particularly in postmenopausal women. It is an important and costly public health problem. Its impact is predicted to escalate dramatically with ageing of the population.

The general principles for medical treatment of osteoporosis are:
- to relieve pain, restore mobility and institute measures to prevent falls
- to exclude and treat underlying diseases that may be responsible for bone fragility
- to establish the severity of osteoporosis by bone densitometry, if this knowledge will influence management
- to stratify the risk of fracture, and decide about therapy (calcium and/or vitamin D supplements, specific osteoporosis therapy, oestrogen/progestin therapy)
- to modify underlying risk factors for fractures.

Drug therapy is aimed at improving bone strength by preventing further bone loss, and/or increasing bone mass:
- Calcium supplementation reduces the rate of bone loss.
- Bisphosphonates slow bone loss and may improve bone mineral density by 4% to 9% over 2 to 3 years, by reducing bone resorption. (Bisphosphonates are also indicated for other bone disease, including Paget's disease, bony metastases, and multiple myeloma. These conditions require higher doses of the more potent nitrogen-containing bisphosphonates [see Box 9, p.76, for different bisphosphonates].)

Dental issues: osteonecrosis of the jaws

Osteonecrosis of the jaws associated with bisphosphonate therapy was first reported in 2003. The risk of osteonecrosis of the jaws associated with bisphosphonate therapy increases with increasing age of the patient, and is greater in those who are medically compromised (particularly those with diabetes and those taking corticosteroids) and those taking nitrogen-containing bisphosphonates (see Box 9 for different bisphosphonates) for malignant bone disease.

Osteonecrosis of the jaws most commonly follows dental extractions, but may be associated with periodontal disease or poorly fitting

---

Box 9. History-taking relating to bisphosphonates

It is highly recommended that dentists check the following points in all medical histories:

1. Do you have any **bone diseases**?

    The conditions which may be treated with bisphosphonates include:
    - osteoporosis
    - Paget's disease
    - cancer with spread to bone (ie breast, prostate, liver, lung and kidney)
    - multiple myeloma
    - other bone conditions

2. Are you taking any **bisphosphonate medications**?

    The commonly prescribed bisphosphonates are:
    - nitrogen-containing bisphosphonates
        - alendronate
        - risedronate
        - disodium pamidronate
        - zoledronic acid
    - non–nitrogen-containing bisphosphonates
        - etidronate
        - sodium clodronate
        - tiludronate

If the patient is at risk of bisphosphonate-associated osteonecrosis (ie the answer to either of the questions is positive), do not proceed to with extraction or surgery without careful establishment of the facts regarding the bone disease and the drug history. Specialist advice may be needed.

Table 7. Risk of osteonecrosis of the jaws in patients taking bisphosphonates*

	Risk of osteonecrosis of the jaws[†]	Risk of osteonecrosis of the jaws if having an extraction[†]
all patients taking bisphosphonates	0.05%–0.10%	0.37%–0.80%
patients with:		
osteoporosis	0.01%–0.04%	0.09%–0.34%
Paget's disease	0.26%–1.8%	2.1%–13.5%
malignancy	0.88%–1.15%	6.67%–9.1%

* This table has been adapted from Mavrokokki A, Cheng A, Stein B, Goss A. The nature and frequency of bisphosphonate associated osteonecrosis of the jaws in Australia. J Oral Maxillofac Surg. In press 2006.
[†] The risk increases with increasing age of patient, increasing time of taking the bisphosphonate, and increasing potency of the bisphosphonate. The risk is higher in patients with immunological compromise (eg corticosteroids, type 1 diabetes).

dentures. It may be apparently spontaneous in onset. The initial Australian experience has been reported in the *Medical Journal of Australia** and the *Australian Dental Journal*.[†] An Australian study[‡] reported the incidence of osteonecrosis of the jaws in patients taking bisphosphonates. The risk of osteonecrosis of the jaws increased with duration of bisphosphonate therapy, the potency of the bisphosphonate, and the total dose. If dental extractions were performed, the calculated incidence was significantly higher. The study differentiated frequencies for patients with osteoporosis, Paget's disease, and malignancy (see Table 7 for results).

Osteonecrosis of the jaws usually involves pain, and there may be obvious exposure of bone in the mouth. Sometimes there is a draining sinus, with extensive undermining of the surrounding mucosa overlying the necrotic bone. The most common complication of osteonecrosis of the jaws is soft tissue infection, which may be extensive.

Dental practitioners must determine whether their patient is at risk of bisphosphonate-associated osteonecrosis (see Box 9 for questions to be asked in the history). If the patient *is* at risk of bisphosphonate-associated osteonecrosis (ie the answer to either of the questions in

---

* Carter G, Goss AN, Doecke C. Bisphosphonates and avascular necrosis of the jaw: a possible association. Med J Aust 2005;182(8):413–5.
† Cheng A, Mavrokokki A, Carter G, Stein B, Fazzalari NL, Wilson DF, et al. The dental implications of bisphosphonates and bone disease. Aust Dent J 2005;50(4 Suppl 2):S4–13.
‡ Mavrokokki A, Cheng A, Stein B, Goss A. The nature and frequency of bisphosphonate associated osteonecrosis of the jaws in Australia. J Oral Maxillofac Surg. In press 2006.

Box 9 is positive), do *not* proceed with extraction or surgery without careful establishment of the facts regarding the bone disease and the drug history. A detailed discussion with the patient is required, and informed consent obtained before extractions or surgery involving bone. Patients with osteoporosis who are medically well can usually be managed in general dental practice. Seriously medically-compromised patients on infused doses of bisphosphonates for malignancy are best managed by a dental specialist associated with the oncology team.

Before commencing bisphosphonate therapy for any patient, a medical practitioner should refer the patient to a dental practitioner to ensure that they are dentally fit and unlikely to require extractions in the foreseeable future.

The medical practitioner should:
- ensure the patient has a proven indication for bisphosphonate therapy
- refer the patient for dental assessment
- commence bisphosphonate therapy (after dental treatment, if required).

The dental practitioner should establish dental fitness:
- eliminate caries (extractions, restorations)
- establish healthy periodontium (scaling, extractions)
- advise the medical practitioner when the patient is dentally fit.

After commencing bisphosphonate therapy, the dental practitioner should monitor oral health regularly, with:
- clinical dental examinations
- radiographs
- dental treatment
  - maintain oral health
  - avoid extractions
  - ensure dentures fit well.

Patients who are taking bisphosphonates should not have extractions or bone surgery until careful assessment of the risk of osteonecrosis of the jaws has been undertaken. Bisphosphonates enter the bone matrix where they remain for at least one, and possibly up to ten, years. The risk of osteonecrosis of the jaws is related to the potency of the bisphosphonate, the dose, and the length of time the patient has been taking the bisphosphonate; the patient's underlying bone condition, age, and concomitant medical conditions are also factors.

The patient must be informed of the risks before deciding whether to proceed to surgery (including extractions). It is important that bisphosphonate therapy is not ceased or changed without consultation with the patient's medical practitioner.

> ***Patients should not cease bisphosphonate therapy without the consent of their medical practitioner.***

All procedures involving bone (eg implant placement, orthodontic tooth movement, periapical or radicular surgery, or root planing) require careful consideration and informed consent before proceeding.* Patients with dental implants who have started taking bisphosphonates need to have their implants monitored as loss of osseointegration may occur.

If an extraction is unavoidable, it should be performed with the minimum of trauma and with direct closure of the socket by suturing. If the patient is medically compromised (particularly if they have diabetes or are taking corticosteroids), consider antibiotic prophylaxis (see pp.140–1).

Monitor the extraction wound until it heals. The healing may be slow; if the socket is still clinically visible at six weeks, specialist advice should be sought, as osteonecrosis of the jaws may have occurred.

Do not curette nonhealing sockets.

An alternative approach to extractions is to exfoliate the tooth using elastic orthodontic bands placed over the crown down onto the root. Usually the tooth will exfoliate over 2 to 4 weeks, particularly if the patient wiggles it. There is little bone exposed by this technique, as the epithelium migrates apically in advance of the elastic band.

Patients with **established osteonecrosis of the jaws** require urgent specialist referral, as they require close long-term monitoring.

> ***Much is unknown about bisphosphonate-associated osteonecrosis of the jaws and its treatment. The above treatment suggestions are not based on formal studies but on best experience to date on this new condition.***

NEUROLOGICAL CONDITIONS

A wide range of neurological conditions may have an impact on dental treatment (eg dementia—an increasing problem in Australia's ageing population—can lead to diagnostic problems and lack of understanding of treatment progress). However, this section discusses only the medication issues associated with neurological conditions related to

---

* *For more information, see position statement on behalf of the Australian and New Zealand Bone and Mineral Society, Osteoporosis Australia, Medical Oncology Group of Australia, and the Australian Dental Association. Bisphosphonates and osteonecrosis of the jaw. Aust Fam Physician 2006(Oct);35(10):801–3.*

stroke, epilepsy and trigeminal neuralgia. These conditions are further discussed in *Therapeutic Guidelines: Neurology*.

Stroke

Stroke is the third most common cause of death in Western countries and the major cause of long-term disability in adults. The current approach to stroke therapy consists of aggressive primary and secondary prevention by control of risk factors.

Primary prevention involves risk-factor management in individuals who have not experienced cerebral vascular symptoms. The risk factors are atrial fibrillation, hypertension, smoking, diabetes, cardiovascular disease and hypercholesterolaemia.

The main medical management used in secondary prevention is antiplatelet therapy. Patients with atrial fibrillation may be taking warfarin. (See pp.62–3 for dental management of patients taking antiplatelet drugs.)

Acute stroke and its management are discussed in 'Medical emergencies' (p.176).

Dental issues

Dental treatment for patients who have had a stroke may need to be modified depending on the patient's medical state and prognosis.

Patients with residual motor defects of the arm, secondary to stroke, may have difficulty cleaning their teeth. Large-handled or electric toothbrushes may improve the effectiveness of oral hygiene.

Patients with seventh cranial (facial) nerve weakness accumulate food debris on the affected side, and may have difficulty with dentures. Design modifications to dentures include a thickened flange. An implant-borne prosthesis may be of benefit, but the patient needs to be able to cope with the additional treatment load, and be able to maintain effective oral hygiene.

Anticoagulants should not be ceased for dentoalveolar procedures but should be managed as outlined in Box 7 (p.64).

Epilepsy

The epilepsies are a group of chronic neurological conditions that are characterised by recurrent unprovoked epileptic seizures. Epilepsy may be the primary problem, or it may be a secondary symptom of some other brain disorder. The epilepsies are best considered as syndromes or diseases which are characterised by the occurrence of one or more seizure types and the presence of associated features. Epileptic seizures may be partial or generalised.

The aim of pharmacotherapy is to maximise the patient's quality of life by preventing seizure recurrence, preferably with monotherapy, and minimising adverse effects. Noncompliance with treatment and with lifestyle advice is a common cause of therapy failure.

Dental issues

The stability of the patient's epilepsy must be assessed—this includes how frequently seizures occur and what triggers them. Before each appointment, check if the patient has taken their medication that day.

> *A person with stable epilepsy who has not taken their medication in the last 12 to 48 hours is potentially at risk of a seizure.*

Avoid stressful extended procedures, which may trigger seizures. Consider the use of a mouth prop, so that if the patient suffers a generalised seizure during treatment, the operator's fingers and instruments can be retrieved.

Some patients develop gingival hyperplasia secondary to antiepilepsy medication. This can be minimised with good oral hygiene. Extensive hyperplasia requires specialist management.

The management of an acute seizure is presented in 'Medical emergencies' (see Box 24, p.177).

Trigeminal neuralgia

Trigeminal neuralgia is characterised by sudden, brief and very severe paroxysms of pain on one side of the face, in the distribution of one or more branches of the fifth cranial (trigeminal) nerve. Because of the very brief nature of the pain, it is sometimes described as stabbing, or compared to an electric shock. Attacks are triggered by trivial sensory stimulation (eg touching the face, cold air blowing on the face, or activities such as talking, chewing, face-washing or toothbrushing). A specific trigger point can sometimes be identified on the gingivae. The pain usually does not awaken the patient from sleep; indeed sleep is a period of relief. There may be a residual ache after the shock-like pain has subsided, but if pain persists at full intensity for more than a few minutes, other diagnoses (eg paroxysmal hemicrania, atypical facial pain) should be considered. Attacks may remit for weeks or months, but then return. There is no sensory loss in the painful area.

Trigeminal neuralgia should be distinguished from post-herpetic neuralgia (where there is a history of herpes zoster eruption). Trigeminal neuralgia in a young person (under 40 years) may be due to multiple sclerosis.

Management of trigeminal neuralgia is primarily by pharmacotherapy (eg carbamazepine).

Dental issues

Many patients who have trigeminal neuralgia think they have toothache and present to the dental practitioner first, or are seen by their medical practitioner and sent to the dentist. Dental pain, particularly pulpitis, is very similar in presentation to trigeminal neuralgia, so careful evaluation of the teeth is required. If the findings from an oral examination and tests (eg pulp tests and radiographs) are inconsistent with the patient's symptoms, do not commence invasive or irreversible procedures. Furthermore, if dental treatment makes no difference to the pain, the possibility of trigeminal neuralgia should be considered before further dental treatment is started. The differences are subtle (but are more evident with careful checking—Is the pain consistent with the condition of the teeth? Can it be stimulated by soft tissue contact? Does it interfere with sleep? What are the effects of diagnostic blocks?).

Nerve blocks with long-acting local anaesthetic (eg bupivacaine with adrenaline) not only give diagnostic information and temporary relief so the patient can eat, but also decrease pain for up to 14 days, thus enhancing the effectiveness of pharmacotherapy.

In patients with unstable trigeminal neuralgia, dental treatment may exacerbate the pain, even if performed on other sites in the mouth. If this occurs, it may help to block the area afflicted by trigeminal neuralgia with a local anaesthetic while treating the other areas; this reduces the degree of exacerbation.

Carbamazepine is an effective analgesic for toothache, so response to carbamazepine is *not* diagnostic of trigeminal neuralgia. The adverse effects of carbamazepine contraindicate its use as a dental analgesic.

If there is uncertainty whether pain is due to a dental problem or to trigeminal neuralgia, the patient requires a specialist referral before the commencement of dental treatment.

If patients with a trigeminal nerve injury from either a local anaesthetic injection or a tooth extraction have a painful dysaesthesic sensory nerve change, they may be helped by medications such as carbamazepine. If such injuries are more than transitory, specialist referral is recommended.

VIRAL DISEASES

Viral hepatitis

Acute viral hepatitis may be caused by hepatitis A, B, C, D and E viruses, and occasionally other viruses. General supportive care forms the basis of treatment, although antiviral therapy may be indicated for hepatitis B and C. For further information on viral hepatitis, see *Therapeutic Guidelines: Gastrointestinal*.

Dental issues

Patients with viral hepatitis B, C or D present a particular challenge to dental practitioners. There are two main principles to prevent transmission:

- All members of the dental team should be vaccinated against hepatitis B.
- All dental practitioners must follow standard precautions with all patients. This is not just for known hepatitis patients (because for every known patient there is at least one who is not known).

Patients with hepatitis C have a higher incidence of dental caries and periodontal disease than age- and sex-matched patients without hepatitis C. Periodontal health in particular is markedly poorer, and salivary flow is reduced. This may be related to lifestyle factors as well as to a direct viral effect. The healing response of the soft tissue to surgery is also poorer.

Dental treatment should be modified in patients with hepatitis C, with a heavy emphasis on preventive care. Patients with advanced dental disease are best treated by extractions, as the response to routine dental treatment is poor. If a patient has advanced hepatitis C or is taking antiviral drugs, antibiotic prophylaxis for high-risk dental procedures (see Table 14, p.137) should be considered (see pp.140–1 for antibiotic prophylaxis regimens).

In general, patients with viral hepatitis should avoid taking sedative and nonsteroidal anti-inflammatory drugs (NSAIDs), as they may be hepatotoxic. Paracetamol-based analgesics can be used sparingly.

Patients may also have issues with excess alcohol consumption or intravenous drug use that may affect compliance with dental treatment.

Needlestick injuries are an uncommon cause of hepatitis B and C. Individual hospitals and health districts have their own infection control policies to deal with such injuries. The principles of these policies are discussed in *Therapeutic Guidelines: Antibiotic*.

Human immunodeficiency virus

Human immunodeficiency virus (HIV) therapeutics is a specialised field, and only practitioners with experience in HIV management should initiate or change antiviral therapy. Patients with symptomatic HIV infection require treatment. Treatment of patients with asymptomatic HIV infection depends on the CD4 count and viral load. Treatment with antiretroviral drugs may significantly delay disease progression.

There are several different groups of antiretroviral drugs—nucleoside/nucleotide reverse transcriptase inhibitors (eg abacavir), non-nucleoside reverse transcriptase inhibitors (eg nevirapine), protease inhibitors (eg ritonavir) and HIV entry inhibitors (eg enfuvirtide). These all have significant drug interactions and potential adverse reactions but the benefits include prolonged life with improved quality.

For further information on HIV infection and its management, see *Therapeutic Guidelines: Antibiotic*.

Dental issues

The prevalence of people living with HIV infection is expected to rise, and those people are increasingly likely to seek care from practitioners who are not specialists in managing HIV. There are changes occurring in the management of HIV infection, and an increase in the number and complexity of antiretroviral regimens. There is the potential for antiretroviral drugs to interact with many commonly prescribed drugs (eg erythromycin, codeine, itraconazole, diazepam), so patients require close monitoring and may need alteration of drug dosage or timing of administration.

Unusual and rare adverse reactions (eg perioral paraesthesia) can occur with antiretroviral drugs.

Consultation with an HIV expert is strongly recommended before starting any new medication for patients taking antiretroviral drugs.

Approximately 50% of patients with HIV/AIDS are smokers. These patients therefore have an increased likelihood of oral diseases such as periodontal disease, leukoplakia, and oral squamous cell carcinoma, so thorough dental examination, treatment and monitoring is required.

HEAD AND NECK CANCER

The morbidity and mortality of head and neck cancer is high. The primary therapeutic management of head and neck cancer is by surgery and/or radiotherapy, sometimes with adjuvant chemotherapy.

A patient with head or neck cancer may be in a weakened state from the effects of both the disease and its treatment. The effects of radiotherapy are localised to the treatment area, whereas chemotherapy affects the whole body.

Dental issues

Dental practitioners have a responsibility in the initial recognition and diagnosis of oropharyngeal cancer. Specialist dental practitioners are an essential part of the head and neck cancer team.

Patients who require head and neck radiotherapy should be reviewed by a dental practitioner experienced in cancer management, to ensure that they are dentally fit and able to maintain their teeth through the oral pain, mucositis and xerostomia that occur with irradiation. If there is doubt that this will be possible, the teeth are best extracted. Radiotherapy can start 7 to 10 days after extractions are completed.

If a patient requires extractions after radiotherapy has been completed, there is a risk of **osteoradionecrosis**. If possible, dental treatment for patients who have had radiotherapy for head and neck cancer should be conservative, by restorations, endodontics and fluoride application. Osteoradionecrosis can be minimised by the use of prophylactic hyperbaric oxygen therapy. Do *not* extract teeth from an irradiated mandible without specialist advice. Usually prophylactic hyperbaric oxygen is required. If prophylactic antibiotics are given alone (without hyperbaric oxygen), they may be insufficient to prevent osteoradionecrosis. Maxillary extractions are generally not a problem, but specialist advice is recommended before proceeding with any extraction. Osteoradionecrosis is painful, seriously debilitating, and difficult to treat. Specialist input is required in the management, which usually requires hyperbaric oxygen in combination with surgical resection of the necrotic bone.

> *In patients who have had oropharyngeal cancer treatment and who present with dental symptoms, the possibility of recurrence of their original cancer or a new primary cancer must be considered and excluded.*

CHEMOTHERAPY

Chemotherapy with cytotoxic drugs is widely used in the management of patients with malignancy. There is a great variety of agents used singly or in combination (sometimes with corticosteroids).

Chemotherapy results in mucositis of the entire gastrointestinal tract. This is commonly the dose-limiting factor of treatment. A similar, but localised, effect occurs with radiotherapy.

Dental issues

Patients should be dentally fit before starting chemotherapy, particularly if the drug regimen will result in severe mucositis and xerostomia.

Dental treatment should be modified to suit the patient's needs and circumstances, and should be performed in the phase between chemotherapy treatments. Dental extraction sockets heal well (and do not have the same problems as those that occur with radiotherapy). Caution is required for patients taking bisphosphonates, and specialist advice should be sought. (See pp.76–9 for information about patients taking bisphosphonates.)

The patient should be warned of the probability of mucositis (and its nature and likely duration) before beginning chemotherapy treatment. The aims of management of mucositis are to reduce pain (using mouthwashes) and to relieve inflammation, so as to enable some oral dietary intake. Patients with mucositis are usually unable to brush their teeth because of pain. (See pp.121–3 for mucositis.)

CHRONIC MUSCULOSKELETAL DISORDERS

Rheumatological diseases encompass arthropathies, myopathies, systemic vasculitis syndromes, and musculoskeletal and connective tissue disorders. Many of these conditions have a degenerative, inflammatory or autoimmune basis, and are chronic and progressive.

Chronic pain problems include chronic back or neck pain, osteoarthritis, rheumatoid arthritis, fibromyalgia, and complex regional pain syndromes.

The management of chronic pain is complex, and includes advice on lifestyle factors, diet and weight control, smoking cessation, and physical activity. Pharmacological management may include the use of analgesics (eg paracetamol, nonsteroidal anti-inflammatory drugs [NSAIDs], opioids), corticosteroids, disease-modifying and immune-modulating antirheumatic drugs, specific drugs for specific conditions (eg allopurinol for gout), and also complementary and alternative medicines.

Dental issues

Dental patients with musculoskeletal problems may find extended dental treatment uncomfortable, and it may exacerbate their medical condition. Modification of treatment to minimise the time spent in the dental chair is recommended. Modifications of the chair configuration and filler pillows to support the neck, hips or knees should be considered.

Some patients have artificial joints. The issues around whether a patient with an artificial joint needs antibiotic prophylaxis are discussed on p.140 and pp.142–3.

Some patients may be taking significant doses of a corticosteroid. The problems with dental treatment in patients taking corticosteroids are discussed on pp.74–5.

Some patients may be taking large doses of analgesics including opioids (narcotics) (either medically directed, or self-obtained in combination with alternative medications or street drugs). Some of these, particularly if taken with tricyclic antidepressants, result in xerostomia (see pp.122–4 for xerostomia).

Temporomandibular disorders

Temporomandibular disorders are musculoskeletal disorders of the masticatory apparatus; these may involve the upper and lower jaws, the masticatory muscles, the temporomandibular joints, the teeth, and the occlusion.

Temporomandibular disorders are commonly misdiagnosed or undiagnosed, and frequently patients are subjected to inappropriate diagnostic and therapeutic procedures. This often leads to considerable patient concern and, as a consequence, the condition can be associated with psychological disturbances, particularly anxiety and depression.

Optimal management initially should be by counselling. Patients should be told about the nature of the disorder and its treatment (which may be prolonged). Discussion should also include the prognosis, which is usually good unless it is complicated by a concurrent psychological disorder. Pain may be relieved by a mild analgesic and the use of warm packs applied to the preauricular region. Patients should be counselled to limit joint function during mastication, speech, occupation, sport and musical instrument playing, as well as limiting parafunctional habits such as clenching, nail-biting or finger-sucking. If their temporomandibular disorder is of short duration (2 to 3 months), approximately two-thirds of patients have resolution of their painful problem and a return to normal function following adequate counselling.

If counselling is not effective, a therapeutic occlusal splint could be considered. This is a hard plastic device worn during sleep on the upper or lower teeth. Splints are presumed to reduce the load on both masticatory muscles and jaw joints, and thereby assist with resolution (much as a crutch reduces load on a sprained ankle). Occlusal splint therapy usually requires six months or more of sleep-time wearing. The splint should be meticulously adjusted for balanced occlusion at approximately monthly intervals during this time. Occlusal splints that are designed to 'reposition' the mandibular condyles are not recommended. Manipulative physiotherapy is not advised in the management of an acutely painful temporomandibular disorder, but gentle massage and gentle exercises may be helpful.

Following the resolution of pain and the return to adequate function, management of occlusal problems, such as by providing adequate dentures or special prostheses (eg overlay dentures) may be necessary. Extensive occlusal rehabilitation with complete crown and bridgework is not recommended.

It is important to differentiate temporomandibular disorder pain from muscular, osteoarthritic, inflammatory and diffuse musculoskeletal pain. It is essential to know if the temporomandibular disorder pain is confined to the jaw or is part of an overall musculoskeletal disorder and/or psychological disorder. Pharmacological management with analgesics (eg nonsteroidal anti-inflammatory [NSAID] drugs) or antidepressant drugs may be part of specialist management.

PSYCHOLOGICAL AND PSYCHIATRIC DISORDERS

Approximately 15% of the population have serious psychological disorders (eg depression) that, if not managed, have major individual and societal consequences. Approximately 2% of the population have a major disorder (eg schizophrenia) which, if untreated, may make it difficult to function in society. Pharmacological treatment is often used in the management of psychological/psychiatric disorders. (See *Therapeutic Guidelines: Psychotropic* for psychiatric conditions and their management.)

Table 8 lists classes of drugs used in psychiatric disorders with some examples of drugs in each class.

Dental issues

The drugs commonly used in dentistry rarely have significant interactions with psychotropic drugs. Local anaesthetics containing adrenaline are

Table 8. Drugs commonly used in psychiatric disorders

Type of drugs	Drug group	Examples of drug
antidepressants	selective serotonin reuptake inhibitors (SSRIs)	fluoxetine, paroxetine
	tricyclic antidepressants (TCAs)	amitriptyline, dothiepin
	monoamine oxidase inhibitors (MAOIs)	phenelzine, moclobemide
mood stabilisers (used in bipolar disorder)		carbamazepine, lamotrigine, lithium, sodium valproate
antipsychotic drugs	typical antipsychotics	haloperidol, trifluoperazine
	atypical antipsychotics	risperidone, olanzapine
psychostimulants		dexamphetamine, methylphenidate, modafinil
anxiolytics and hypnotics	benzodiazepines	diazepam, temazepam
	others	zolpidem, zopiclone
antiparkinsonian drugs		benztropine, benzhexol
drugs used in alcohol and drug disorders		methadone, naltrexone
drugs used in dementia	cholinesterase inhibitors	rivastigmine
	others	memantine

not contraindicated with tricyclic antidepressants and selective serotonin reuptake inhibitors (SSRIs). Monoamine oxidase inhibitors (MAOIs) are used less commonly than previously; they have adverse interactions with many medications. Local anaesthetics without adrenaline can be used in patients taking MAOIs, but dental local anaesthetics containing adrenaline are best avoided, as they may interact adversely.

The patient medication list may be helpful in determining the patient's underlying mental health condition.

Examples:

A patient who says they are well but are taking lithium does, in fact, have a serious underlying psychiatric disorder. This knowledge can help define an appropriate treatment plan.

> A patient who has body dysmorphic disorder (which is characterised by a preoccupation with imagined or slight defects in physical appearance) may at first seem an ideal patient for an aesthetic dental procedure; however, no matter how the appearance of their teeth and jaws improves, they will never be satisfied.

Dental practitioners must be aware of the psychological status of their patients, and interactions of the practitioner and the staff with the patient must be appropriate.

Patients with anxiety or phobic states can be difficult to manage; many simply do not present to the dental practitioner for routine treatment and arrive only when a painful emergency occurs. Routine sedatives may be ineffective as the patient might be intolerant to them. General anaesthesia or specialist referral may be required.

Drug-dependent and drug-seeking patients may present to a dental practice. Suspicion should be raised if a patient demands analgesic drugs and exhibits a good level of knowledge or a preference for a particular opioid (narcotic). Do not initiate treatment in the absence of demonstrable disease. Advise the patient to see their medical practitioner—often they will state that they do not attend a practitioner regularly, or that they use several health centres. If you are unable to diagnose a dental condition causing the pain, do *not* give a prescription for an analgesic. At most, offer a small amount of analgesic and direct the patient to consult their medical practitioner.

Drug-dependent and drug-seeking patients are not uncommon in general dental practice.

FURTHER READING

eTG complete [CD-ROM]. Melbourne: Therapeutic Guidelines Limited [regularly updated].

Little JW, Falace DA, Miller CS, Rhodus NL. Dental management of the medically compromised patient. 6th ed. St Louis: Mosby; 2002.

Dental caries

Dental caries (tooth decay) is a pathological process resulting in localised destruction of tooth tissue. The disease begins with the demineralisation of tooth hard tissue by organic acids. Bacteria resident in dental plaque produce these acids by fermenting the carbohydrate in food. (See Figure 2, p.128, for a schematic illustration of tooth infections and caries.) The incidence of dental caries has declined in most developed countries over the last two to three decades because of the use of fluorides; however, the decline in the incidence has now plateaued. The disease is still a major worldwide public health problem.

Dental plaque must be present for caries to develop. Plaque is a complex biofilm, which includes a mixed community of bacteria and their by-products. These bacteria have variable capacities to produce organic acids (eg acetic, lactic and formic acids) from fermentable carbohydrates (particularly dietary sugars). Many bacteria can produce organic acids from fermentable carbohydrates, and frequent exposure to fermentable carbohydrates leads to an increase in the population of cariogenic bacteria (eg *Streptococcus mutans* and *Lactobacillus* species) in the biofilm. These bacteria readily survive in an acid environment and are prolific producers of organic acids, particularly lactic acid. They cause demineralisation because they produce acid at around pH 5, which is below the critical pH range for maintaining the saturation of apatite in the enamel. Enamel demineralisation is caused by an imbalance in the equilibrium between enamel apatite and the calcium, phosphate, and hydroxide ions in the surrounding biofilm fluid. Frequent exposure of the plaque to fermentable carbohydrates maintains the plaque pH below the critical pH for extended periods leading to subsurface enamel demineralisation and the formation of 'white spot' lesions. These lesions have a relatively intact surface, but continued demineralisation can progress to cavitation. The disease is progressive if not treated, leading to larger and deeper cavities. Once cavitation occurs within dentine, the caries gradually progresses towards the dental pulp, and ultimately, if untreated, pulpitis (inflammation of the dental pulp) develops. Once pulpitis is established, pain is experienced with various stimuli. Eventually, if the caries is still untreated, the pulp inflammation will be followed by pulp necrosis and infection of the root canal system; this will then cause inflammation of the periapical tissues (known as apical periodontitis), which can present with a variety of symptoms. Infection of the root canal system can also give rise to spreading infections (see pp.129–32 for spreading infection).

The ability of plaque bacteria to demineralise the tooth surface can be modified by several factors, including:

- diet—patterns of consumption (frequency), and types of diet (eg high sugar)
- plaque composition—the level of cariogenic bacteria in plaque and their capacity to produce a sustained low pH environment
- saliva composition and characteristics (eg flow, buffering capacity, antimicrobial factors, and calcium, phosphate, hydroxide and fluoride ion levels)
- tooth resistance (eg exposure to remineralising agents such as topical fluorides and casein phosphopeptide stabilised amorphous calcium phosphate [CPP-ACP]).

TREATMENT

In the early stages of caries, before cavitation, several strategies can be used:

- plaque reduction by cleaning of teeth
    - brushing at least twice a day with a fluoride toothpaste
    - flossing, preferably immediately before brushing with the toothpaste
    - use of other interdental cleaning aids
- dietary modification, particularly the avoidance of sucrose in sticky forms or as sweet snacks between meals
- plaque modification by reducing the level of cariogenic bacteria in plaque by using antimicrobial products (eg chlorhexidine gel) or the antibacterial effect of topical fluoride at high concentrations and in an acidulated form
- tooth surface modification by the application of remineralising agents such as fluorides and casein phosphopeptide stabilised amorphous calcium phosphate (CPP-ACP), and by the placement of fissure sealants
- increased salivary flow and function by using sugar-free chewing gum or nonacidic coarse foods (eg carrots).

After cavitation, the caries must be removed and the cavity restored; however, strategies must still be used to prevent further decay.

Table 9 (p.95) shows examples of topical applications and how they can be used for caries reduction.

Fluoride

In randomised controlled clinical trials, the use of fluoride-containing toothpastes and mouthwashes significantly reduced the incidence of caries. The efficacy of these products in reducing caries activity has been attributed to their ability to incorporate fluoride ions into plaque, as several studies have shown an inverse relationship between plaque fluoride concentrations and caries. Fluoride ions in plaque immediately promote the formation of fluorhydroxyapatite and/or fluorapatite in the presence of the calcium and phosphate ions produced during enamel demineralisation by plaque acids.

When the fluoride ion promotes remineralisation, it forms fluorhydroxyapatite or fluorapatite instead of hydroxyapatite. These fluoride-containing apatites are more resistant to future acid challenge. Fluoride ions at very high concentrations and low pH (eg acidulated phosphate fluoride) also have some antimicrobial activity as hydrofluoric acid crosses the bacterial cell membrane and inhibits the organism's metabolism.

Care needs to be taken with fluoride toothpastes and other forms of fluoride used by children younger than 6 years of age, to minimise ingestion of fluoride and the risk of dental fluorosis. Children younger than 18 months should have their teeth cleaned with a soft toothbrush, but with *no* toothpaste. For children between the age of 18 months and 6 years, toothpaste with 400 to 550 ppm (parts per million) fluoride ion should be used under the supervision of a responsible adult. A small pea-sized amount of toothpaste should be applied to a child-sized soft toothbrush. Children should spit out and not swallow the toothpaste.

Community water fluoridation is supported by scientific evidence as an effective, inexpensive and safe community health measure.

There are a number of additional ways to apply fluoride (see Table 9, p.95).

Fluoride supplements in the form of drops or tablets are no longer recommended because of the risk of fluorosis.

In the early 1990s, when fluoride supplements were still recommended and before the introduction of 400 to 550 ppm fluoride toothpastes (ie a lower dose than for adults) for children younger than 6 years of age, the prevalence of dental fluorosis was unacceptably high. However, since the introduction of low-fluoride toothpaste for children and the phasing out of fluoride supplements (which are no longer recommended), the prevalence of fluorosis has declined.

All persons over 18 months of age can benefit from using fluoridated toothpaste. After brushing, the toothpaste should be spat out and not swallowed; the mouth should not be rinsed:

children 18 months to 5 years (inclusive)—fluoride toothpaste 400 to 550 ppm (0.4–0.55 mg/g), a pea-sized amount, twice daily

adults and children 6 years and over—fluoride toothpaste 1000 ppm (1 mg/g) twice daily.

Table 9 shows examples of topical fluoride applications and how they can be used for caries reduction in patients at risk of caries.

Chlorhexidine

Chlorhexidine mouthwashes are commonly used for a short time to help reduce levels of supragingival dental plaque in adults.

Chlorhexidine gel is preferred for caries control as it has fewer adverse effects than the mouthwash and it can be used once a week. (See p.59 for more information about chlorhexidine.) Chlorhexidine has a role in caries-susceptible children and adults. The anionic detergent sodium lauryl sulphate used in standard toothpaste inactivates chlorhexidine, so chlorhexidine should not be used immediately before or after using a standard toothpaste.

Table 9 shows examples of topical applications and how they can be used for caries reduction.

Casein phosphopeptide stabilised amorphous calcium phosphate (CPP-ACP)

Calcium ions and phosphate ions are required with fluoride ions for the formation of fluorapatite. In the normal mouth, the availability of calcium and phosphate ions can be limiting for fluoride's action, and this is exacerbated in a dry mouth. Calcium and phosphate ions cannot be easily applied intraorally as they rapidly combine into insoluble forms where the ions are not bioavailable. A new form of calcium phosphate has been developed whereby the calcium and phosphate ions are held in a bioavailable form using phosphopeptides from the milk protein casein. This form of calcium phosphate, referred to as casein phosphopeptide stabilised amorphous calcium phosphate (CPP-ACP), can help to slow the progression of caries and promote the regression of early stages of the disease. CPP-ACP is available in a sugar-free chewing gum and in a professionally applied cream (see Table 9).

Table 9. Examples of topical applications and how they may be used for caries reduction in patients at elevated risk of developing caries

Application	Example of how application may be used*
fluoride	
fluoride varnish 22 600 ppm (22.6 mg/mL)	Apply in the dental surgery to all at-risk dental surfaces at the clinician's discretion, usually twice a year.
acidulated phosphate fluoride gel or foam 1500–12 300 ppm (1.5–12.3 mg/g)	Can be used by people aged 10 years or more. Apply in the dental surgery for 4 minutes using trays. (Evacuate excess, and spit out residual gel after tray removal.) Adults can use the gel daily at home, or apply it using customised trays. (Acidulated gel or foam is preferred as it has better enamel uptake; however, it is better to use neutral gel or foam in patients with porcelain restorations and those undergoing head and/or neck irradiation.)
fluoride rinse 200–1000 ppm (0.2–1 mg/mL)	Can be used daily by people aged 6 years or more. After rinsing, the mouthwash should be spat out and not swallowed.
neutral fluoride toothpaste 5000 ppm (5 mg/g)	Use daily in adults with a high risk of caries.
chlorhexidine	
chlorhexidine 0.2% gel	Brush on the teeth (pea-sized amount on a soft toothbrush) either once a week or daily for 7–14 days.
casein phosphopeptide stabilised amorphous calcium phosphate (CPP-ACP)	
CPP-ACP sugar-free gum	Can be used 4 times daily, preferably after meals and after cleaning teeth with a fluoride toothpaste.
CPP-ACP cream	Apply professionally after dental procedures and after topical fluoride applications. Adults with an elevated risk of developing caries can apply nightly to teeth after tooth-cleaning and not rinse out.

* The decision is based on clinical judgment and requires a complete assessment of the patient (eg age, other medications, disease risk).

FURTHER READING

Australian Research Centre for Population Oral Health, Dental School, The University of Adelaide, South Australia. The use of fluorides in Australia: guidelines. Aust Dent J 2006;51(2):195–9.

Fejerskov O, Kidd E, editors. Dental caries: the disease and its clinical management. 2nd ed. Oxford: Blackwell Munksgaard; 2003.

Kidd E, Joyston-Bechal S. Essentials of dental caries: the disease and its management. 2nd ed. Oxford: Oxford University Press; 1997.

Thylstrup A, Fejerskov O, editors. Textbook of clinical cariology. 2nd ed. Copenhagen: Munksgaard; 1994.

Periodontal disease

Periodontal disease is inflammation of the gingivae and the supporting structures of the teeth—the periodontal ligament, the cementum and the alveolar bone. The most common forms of periodontal disease present as chronic conditions. There are two major forms of chronic periodontal diseases—plaque-induced gingivitis (below) and periodontitis (p.98). Periodontitis has two major variations—chronic and aggressive. Acute forms of periodontal disease include acute ulcerative gingivitis (p.99) and periodontal abscess (p.100).

Periodontal disease is caused by dental plaque—a complex biofilm of microorganisms and their by-products that builds up on the teeth. Plaque can calcify to become calculus. The accumulation of plaque and calculus is associated with poor oral hygiene; that is, the teeth have not been cleaned thoroughly and/or often enough.

In the early stage of periodontal disease, bacteria in plaque cause inflammation of the gingivae—gingivitis. Gingivitis can usually be treated successfully by removal of the plaque and calculus followed by thorough and regular oral hygiene practices. In some patients, untreated gingivitis progresses to a more advanced stage of periodontal disease called 'periodontitis', which may result in loss of the bone and the tissues that support the teeth. As gingival inflammation progresses, periodontal pockets are formed, and the gingivae may recede from the teeth. As a result of damage to the supporting tissues, the teeth can become loose, and may eventually exfoliate or require extraction. (See Figure 2, p.128, for locations of infections around the tooth.)

GINGIVITIS

Gingivitis is inflammation restricted to the gingival tissues, which become red and swollen, and bleed easily. It is rarely painful and, with correct treatment, is reversible. Gingivitis develops because of the presence of an undisturbed bacterial biofilm (plaque) in the gingival crevices and adjacent to the gingival margins. The gingival inflammation caused by this biofilm is a nonspecific inflammatory response to the diffusion of bacterial antigenic products into the adjacent gingival tissue.

Management

Gingivitis should be managed by a dentist. The aim of the treatment is to remove plaque (by thorough dental cleaning) and smooth any roughness on the teeth (eg calculus) that allows plaque to accumulate. This should be combined with patient education about oral hygiene. Calculus deposits are removed by dental scaling (eg ultrasonic cleaning and/or hand scaling). Complete resolution of the inflammation can be expected within one week.

The short-term use of a mouthwash to inhibit supragingival plaque formation may be useful when inflammation restricts normal brushing:

> *chlorhexidine 0.2% mouthwash*, 10 mL rinsed in the mouth for 1 minute, 8- to 12-hourly for 5 to 10 days*
> *or chlorhexidine 0.12% mouthwash*, 15 mL rinsed in the mouth for 1 minute, 8- to 12-hourly for 5 to 10 days.*

PERIODONTITIS

Periodontitis is inflammation affecting the periodontal ligament, gingiva, cementum and alveolar bone, resulting in loss of tooth support with progressive bone loss and, ultimately, loose teeth. There may be pocket formation and/or gingival recession. It is often associated with oral malodour and bad taste. In advanced cases, the teeth may drift, allowing spaces to develop between the teeth.

Major risk factors for the development and progression of periodontitis include smoking and poorly controlled diabetes.

Usually the disease presents in a chronic slowly progressing form (with brief acute episodes). However, a relatively aggressive form may present; this requires specialist management.

Periodontitis is rarely seen in children. Children require urgent specialist review because periodontitis in children is almost invariably associated with systemic disease.

Management

The management of periodontitis requires debridement to break up the biofilm. Systemic antibiotics are not effective without debridement, as they cannot penetrate the biofilm.

Treatment protocols include:
- thorough **toothbrushing** and **interdental cleaning**

---

* *With prolonged use (more than a few days), chlorhexidine may cause a superficial discolouration of the teeth and fillings (see p.59 for more information).*

- **patient education** about oral hygiene and habit management, particularly smoking cessation
- removal of calculus and plaque with **dental scaling** (eg ultrasonic cleaning or hand scaling)
- **root planing (debridement)**, which involves removal of calculus and plaque from deeper pockets, together with planing of the roots. This is often done under local anaesthetic and is usually accompanied by polishing, reshaping, or replacement of defective fillings
- in advanced periodontal disease, **periodontal surgery**, which involves raising a mucoperiosteal flap to assist root planing, may be necessary and is sometimes associated with bone recontouring.

Antibiotic therapy is rarely required, and is not effective without concomitant debridement.

Unresponsive or aggressive periodontal disease and periodontitis in an immunocompromised patient should be managed by a specialist.

ACUTE ULCERATIVE GINGIVITIS

Acute ulcerative gingivitis (previously known as acute necrotising ulcerative gingivitis [ANUG], trench mouth, and Vincent's disease) is an extremely painful infection of the periodontal tissues. It is characterised by punched-out interdental papillae, ulcers (often covered with a greyish membrane) and, usually, a fetid odour. It is rarely associated with systemic signs and symptoms.

Acute ulcerative gingivitis is most commonly seen in young adult smokers. It is rarely seen in children. In children, acute herpetic gingivostomatitis (see pp.115–16) is sometimes misdiagnosed as acute ulcerative gingivitis.

Treatment considerations include irrigation and debridement of the necrotic area and tooth surfaces, oral hygiene instruction, oral rinses, pain control, and management of systemic manifestations including appropriate antibiotic therapy, as necessary.

Local debridement (scaling and root planing) is required to stop recurrence. This often cannot be completely performed until lesions become less painful.

The initial management of acute ulcerative gingivitis is usually local debridement (scaling and root planing) under local anaesthesia accompanied by improved plaque control (often with the adjunctive use of chlorhexidine mouthwash), smoking cessation counselling and metronidazole (when systemic signs and symptoms are present). Use:

> *metronidazole 400 mg (child: 10 mg/kg up to 400 mg) orally, 12-hourly for 5 days*
>
> *PLUS*
>
> *chlorhexidine 0.2% mouthwash*, 10 mL rinsed in the mouth for 1 minute, 8- to 12-hourly*
> *or chlorhexidine 0.12% mouthwash*, 15 mL rinsed in the mouth for 1 minute, 8- to 12-hourly.*

Metronidazole is often given as 200 mg orally 3 times daily; however, in these guidelines it is recommended as a 12-hourly regimen, which is thought to increase patient adherence to treatment.

> ***Antibiotic therapy alone, without debridement and oral hygiene improvement, will invariably lead to recurrence.***

In more severe or unresponsive cases specialist referral is indicated.

In patients with HIV infection, acute ulcerative gingivitis can spread to involve the underlying bone (necrotising ulcerative periodontitis) and should be treated by a specialist.

PERIODONTAL ABSCESS

A periodontal abscess is seen almost exclusively in patients with existing periodontal disease and/or uncontrolled diabetes. The discomfort associated with the swelling is usually not enough to keep the patient awake at night. Pain is often difficult to localise. The flora associated with periodontal abscesses is more mixed than with most other periodontal infections. (See Figure 2, p.128, for the locations of infections around the tooth.)

Treatment requires direct mechanical/surgical access to clean the tooth roots of any plaque and calculus. In advanced cases, extractions may be considered.

If systemic signs and symptoms are present, or if the patient is not responding to local treatment (see pp.98–9), antimicrobial therapy should be considered:

1 *phenoxymethylpenicillin 500 mg (child: 10 mg/kg up to 500 mg) orally, 6-hourly for 5 days*

  OR

---

* *With prolonged use (more than a few days), chlorhexidine may cause a superficial discolouration of the teeth and fillings (see p.59 for more information).*

2. *amoxycillin 500 mg (child: 10 mg/kg up to 500 mg) orally, 8-hourly for 5 days*

    OR (for patients hypersensitive to penicillins)

3. *clindamycin 300 mg (child: 7.5 mg/kg up to 300 mg) orally, 8-hourly for 5 days.*

Patients who are not responding to treatment and who wish to retain their teeth require management by a specialist.

FURTHER READING

Carranza FA, Newman MG, editors. Clinical periodontology. 8th ed. Philadelphia: WB Saunders Co; 1996.

Halitosis

Halitosis, or oral malodour, is common on awakening, usually as a result of low salivary flow and lack of oral cleansing during sleep. This rarely has any special significance, and can be readily rectified by eating, tongue-brushing, and rinsing the mouth with fresh water. Halitosis at times other than upon waking usually results from eating various foods (such as garlic, onion or spices), or from habits such as smoking or drinking alcohol. The cause of halitosis is therefore often obvious, and can be prevented by avoiding these substances and habits.

Studies have shown that specific bacteria (*Veillonella*, *Actinomyces* and *Prevotella*) are the predominant producers of hydrogen sulfide (H_2S), and that an increase in the number of these H_2S-producing bacteria in the tongue biofilm is responsible for halitosis. *In vitro* studies modelling the bacterial colonisation of the tongue have shown that although the number of H_2S-producing organisms is low (at about 2.5% of all tongue flora organisms), a reduction in these organisms will decrease the amount of volatile sulfur compounds and thus halitosis. The dorsal surface of the tongue is thought to be the location of the microbial population causing this halitosis. Thus, dental plaque and food debris associated with poor oral hygiene or a poorly designed denture or bridge only *add* to the level of halitosis.

Common causes of halitosis are shown in Box 10 (p.104).

MANAGEMENT

Management of halitosis includes:
- confirming the patient's subjective halitosis (ie noted by family/friends and clinician)
- identifying the cause (which is often multifactorial)
- discussing the condition with the patient (outlining that this is often a controllable rather than a curable condition)
- developing a treatment strategy
- checking compliance and level of success by follow-up.

> **Box 10. Some common causes of halitosis**
>
> Infections within the mouth including:
> - caries
> - dental abscess
> - oral candidosis
> - tonsillitis
>
> Periodontal disease
>
> Mucosal ulcerative conditions
>
> Dry mouth (xerostomia)
>
> Oral cancer
>
> Starvation
>
> Odour-causing foods (eg garlic, onions)
>
> Smoking and drugs (eg alcohol, isosorbide dinitrate)
>
> Poor dental hygiene (eg putrescent food particles between the teeth, on the tongue and around the gums)
>
> Systemic disease (eg hepatic encephalopathy, diabetic acidosis, uraemia, trimethylaminuria, infectious or neoplastic disease of the respiratory or gastrointestinal tract)
>
> Psychogenic factors

Initial management of halitosis requires identifying the cause and assessing the severity of the malodour. Examination of the nose, tonsils, mucosal surfaces of the pharynx and oral cavity, and dentition is required.

Diagnosis of halitosis is usually subjective, by simply smelling exhaled air coming from the patient's mouth and nose and comparing the two. Odour originating in the mouth, but not detectable from the nose is likely to be of oral or pharyngeal origin. Odour originating in the nose may come from the sinuses or nasal passages. Similar odour equally sensed from both the nose and the mouth can indicate one of the many systemic causes. A halimeter is a specific apparatus for objectively measuring the responsible volatile sulfur compounds; however, measurements given by this equipment are variable and the results are difficult to interpret.

Defined infective processes that can cause malodour include periodontal infections, pericoronitis (soft tissue infection associated with a partially erupted tooth), any oral infection (including infected extraction sockets) and mucosal ulcerative conditions (eg recurrent aphthous stomatitis, oral lichen planus). Improvement of oral hygiene, prevention or treatment of infective processes, and sometimes the use of antimicrobials can usually manage this type of halitosis. A mouthwash containing chlorhexidine may be effective in the short-term management of halitosis caused by oral conditions:

> *chlorhexidine 0.2% mouthwash*, 10 mL held in the mouth for 1 minute, 8- to 12-hourly.*

Limited studies have shown that lozenges containing low levels of zinc may reduce the amount of volatile sulfur compounds; other studies have shown that triclosan, a lipid-soluble antibacterial agent, may reduce the amount of volatile sulfur compounds in a dose-dependant fashion. However, neither of these agents has been studied in patients with halitosis.

An occasional clinical dilemma is the complaint of halitosis by patients who do not have it but imagine it. Objective testing is difficult and often unreliable, and the halitosis may then be attributable to a form of delusion or monosymptomatic hypochondriasis (ie psychogenic halitosis). Other people's behaviour, or perceived behaviour, such as covering the nose or averting the face, is typically misinterpreted by these patients as being an indication that their breath is indeed offensive. Such patients may have latent psychosomatic illness. They present a diagnostic and treatment difficulty, and despite reassurance may require psychiatric consultation.

For patients with persistent or recurrent halitosis, a full assessment of oral and dental health by a dental practitioner is advised. If this proves unhelpful, referral for specialist opinion is needed. This may include referral to an oral medicine specialist; an otorhinolaryngologist to rule out the presence of chronic tonsillitis or chronic sinusitis; a physician to rule out gastric, hepatic, endocrine, pulmonary, metabolic or renal disease; and/or a psychologist or psychiatrist.

FURTHER READING

Scully C, Felix DH. Oral medicine—update for the dental practitioner: oral malodour. Br Dent J 2005;199(8):498–500.

---

* *With prolonged use (more than a few days), chlorhexidine may cause a superficial discolouration of the teeth and fillings (see p.59 for more information).*

Oral mucosal disease

Oral inflammatory lesions are common. They can be the result of local disease, a manifestation of cutaneous or gastrointestinal disease, or a sign of systemic disease.

Diagnosis of oral mucosal lesions is made with a full history (including a medication history), a thorough oral examination and, often, cytological, haematological/serological and histopathological investigation. It is important to also examine the skin of patients presenting with oral mucosal disease, as cutaneous diseases can affect the oral mucosa as the presenting complaint (eg pemphigus vulgaris) or as the most persistent complaint (eg lichen planus).

Smears of the oral mucosa are particularly helpful when stained by the periodic acid–Schiff reaction for the presence of fungal hyphae (it is important that antifungal treatment has not been used recently). Fresh tissue, taken as part of the biopsy procedure and placed in isotonic saline or specific transport media (eg Michel's medium, available on request from pathology laboratories), allows the localisation of antigens and antibodies via direct immunofluorescence. This significantly improves the likelihood of a specific diagnosis of an oral mucosal disease.

Mucosal diseases can be divided into three broad sections—mucosal discolourations, ulcerative conditions, and fungal infections. Oral mucositis and xerostomia are also discussed in this chapter.

The management of oral mucosal disease is principally by the use of topical agents. The majority of these agents used intraorally are antiseptic/anaesthetic preparations. Symptomatic relief with these preparations *is* important, but does not alter the underlying disease process, and the use of them alone in most cases represents a significant undertreatment of a (usually) readily manageable condition. The addition of a topical corticosteroid addresses the immune mechanisms responsible for the condition and, with appropriate titration to an individual patient's needs and responsiveness, can be a major step in minimising the often significant functional morbidity associated with recurrent oral ulceration.

MUCOSAL DISCOLOURATIONS

Changes in the oral mucosa can result in a range of discolourations and textural changes. The most common are white patches, which can be manifestations of physiological states—and therefore normal—(eg Fordyce's spots, leukoedema) or pathological states. Pathological states include keratosis (eg idiopathic, frictional, or associated with smoking), epithelial dysplasia, carcinoma, and dermatoses (eg lichen planus).

Leukoplakia

The term 'leukoplakia' refers to a white patch or plaque that cannot be removed and cannot be characterised clinically (or histologically) as any other pathology. See Photo 1 for an example of leukoplakia.

Homogenous leukoplakias tend to be smooth white plaques; they have a malignant transformation rate of about 3%.

Nonhomogenous leukoplakias (including speckled leukoplakias) present as white patches on a red background and have a higher risk of malignant change—about 4 to 5 times that of homogenous leukoplakias (ie up to 15%). Any type of surface irregularity or textural variation always places a white patch into the nonhomogenous category.

The site of leukoplakias is important—leukoplakias on the floor of the mouth and the ventral surface of the tongue have higher rates of malignant transformation. The size of leukoplakias is not significant,

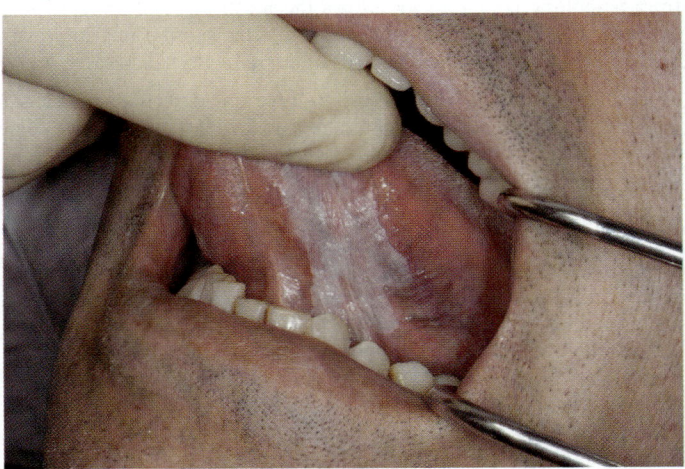

Photo 1. Leukoplakia of the ventral surface of the tongue and floor of mouth

with small and large white lesions equally likely to transform. Other features relating to malignant transformation are duration of the lesion and the use of alcohol and tobacco. If there is doubt about the diagnosis of a white patch, specialist referral is indicated to rule out the possibility of squamous cell carcinoma (see Photo 2).

> *Biopsy of any persistent undiagnosed white oral patch is essential to exclude epithelial dysplasia, carcinoma in situ and squamous cell carcinoma.*

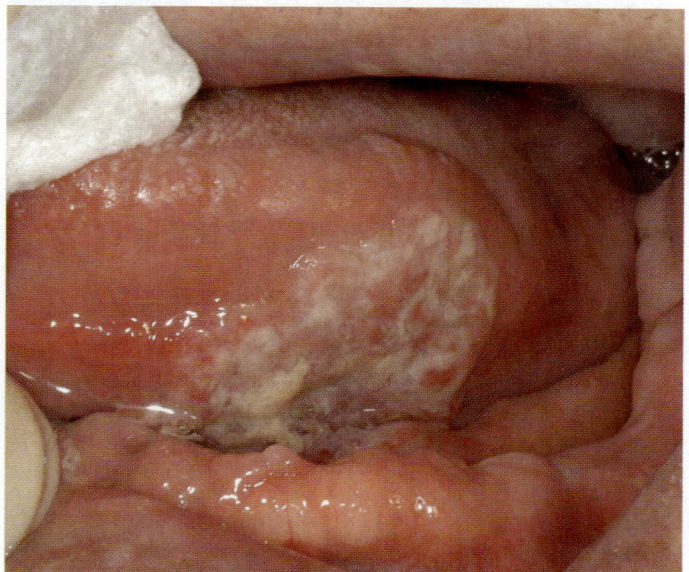

Photo 2. Squamous cell carcinoma of the left lateral margin of the tongue

Oral lichen planus

Lichen planus (see Photo 3, p.110) is an immunologically mediated disease in which T-cells are directed against basal keratinocytes, causing an inflammatory mucositis with characteristic features. The mouth is affected frequently, with lesions typically occurring on the buccal mucosa, tongue and gingivae. In the non-erosive form of the disease, the lesions consist of a characteristic pattern of white striations or plaques. Erosive oral lichen planus presents as erythematous, ulcerated or eroded areas of mucosa, which are often painful. Oral lesions can be persistent, difficult to treat, and can occur in the absence of cutaneous lesions.

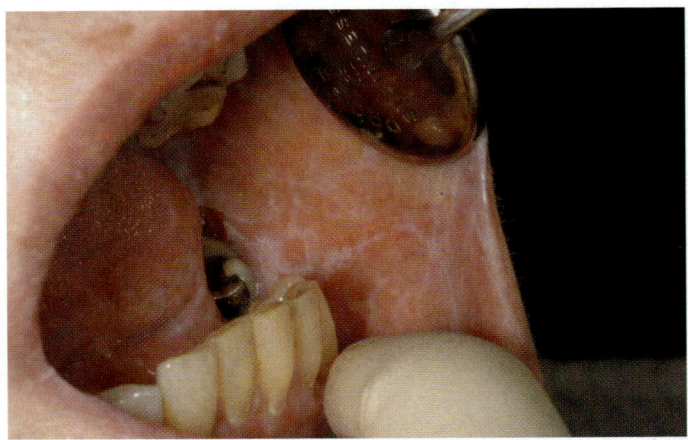

Photo 3. Oral lichen planus of the left buccal mucosa showing white striations

There is a slightly elevated risk of the development of oral squamous cell carcinoma, particularly in erosive forms of lichen planus. Stopping smoking and regular periodic review is strongly recommended.

Most oral lichen planus is idiopathic, although in some cases lichenoid changes of the mucosa are drug-induced, with a wide range of medications being implicated. Dental amalgam restorations have been implicated in rare cases of persistent lichenoid lesions, particularly if the lesions are in close proximity to the amalgam fillings. Hypersensitivity to amalgam can cause an oral lichenoid eruption that mimics idiopathic lichen planus. Patch-testing for any mercury or dental alloy hypersensitivity may be performed to assess patients for specific allergies.

Management

If biopsy-proven oral lichen planus becomes symptomatic, it can be treated with:

1. *triamcinolone acetonide 0.1% paste topically to the lesions, 3 times daily after meals*

    OR

2. *betamethasone dipropionate 0.05% ointment topically to the lesions, 3 times daily after meals*

    OR

3. beclomethasone dipropionate 50 micrograms sprayed on the lesions, 3 times daily after meals.

Topical corticosteroids should not be used continuously for more than six weeks.

If resolution has not occurred within six weeks, specialist consultation should be sought. Treatment may include intralesional corticosteroid, or systemic (oral) prednis(ol)one, particularly if the oral lichen planus is associated with severe cutaneous lichen planus.

Recent studies have introduced a number of newer immunosuppressive drugs (eg topical tacrolimus) that may be effective in controlling symptoms related to oral lichen planus. Further investigation is required to determine if tacrolimus or pimecrolimus is an appropriate treatment for oral lichen planus, but current data are promising for at least some patients with severe and refractory disease.

Geographic tongue

Geographic tongue (erythema migrans) is a benign condition with an incidence of up to 5% in the general population. It manifests as migratory areas of erythema usually involving the dorsal surface of the tongue, but it may extend to the floor of the mouth and even the buccal mucosa. The erythematous areas represent a central atrophic and depapillated zone which, in the most frequently seen pattern, is surrounded by elevated white or cream margins. Occasionally the central erythematous areas are sensitive. Histological examination shows epithelial thinning with an inflammatory infiltrate in the centre of the lesion. Although the cause is unknown, there may be a family history of the condition, and some patients have atopic allergies or can relate the lesions to particular foods or stress. It is occasionally seen in patients with psoriasis; however, it is not associated with any specific condition.

Treatment of geographic tongue is generally not required. If there is pain or burning, specialist consultation is required, as it may be a symptom of 'burning mouth syndrome'.

Hairy tongue

Hairy tongue (usually black, but may be other colours) occurs when excessively long filiform papillae of the tongue become stained by an accumulation of epithelial cells, exogenous material and, perhaps, chromogenic microorganisms. It occurs most commonly with the use of chlorhexidine mouthwash, or after a course of antibiotics. It is also seen in patients who have limited oral intake (eg with percutaneous endoscopic gastrostomy [PEG] feeding).

The main aim of treatment is to identify and eliminate causative factors. In addition, improving oral hygiene, brushing the tongue with a toothbrush and using oxygenating mouthwashes (eg sodium bicarbonate) can help.

Oral hairy leukoplakia

Oral hairy leukoplakia (see Photo 4) usually presents as a fixed white 'corrugated' lesion on the lateral border of the tongue. It can extend onto the dorsal and ventral surfaces of the tongue and to the buccal mucosa. The lesion is associated with Epstein-Barr virus and develops in patients who are immunosuppressed—for example, in patients with HIV infection. It has also been reported to occur in renal transplant recipients.

Generally, oral hairy leukoplakia is asymptomatic; however, some patients complain of a 'burning' sensation, which is often due to secondary infection with *Candida*. Treatment with appropriate antifungal drugs (see p.119) usually resolves the symptoms. Treatment of oral hairy leukoplakia *per se* is not useful, and management must address the underlying immunosuppression.

In the context of HIV infection, the development of oral hairy leukoplakia may indicate increasing HIV viral load, although this is not a reliable diagnostic sign and further investigation may be warranted.

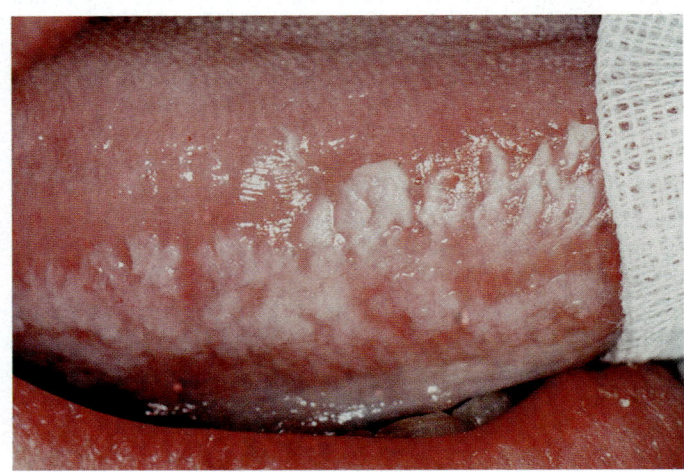

Photo 4. Oral hairy leukoplakia of the right lateral margin of the tongue

ULCERATIVE CONDITIONS

Mouth ulceration most commonly occurs as a result of trauma from eating rough, sharp or hot foods, or from sharp broken teeth or dental fillings. Other important causes are listed in Table 10 (p.114).

Mouth ulcers can be classified into several broad groups—traumatic (see Photo 5), infective (usually viral, occasionally bacterial or fungal), dermatological, neoplastic, and other (including aphthous).

As the predominant cause of oral ulceration is traumatic, the initial management must deal with possible trauma. Management of minor trauma may include changing oral hygiene practices, adjusting appliances, smoothing sharp edges of teeth or restorations, or placing wax on orthodontic appliances.

Ulcers persisting for longer than three weeks are potentially neoplastic; patients with such ulcers require specialist input into their management, and biopsy should be considered.

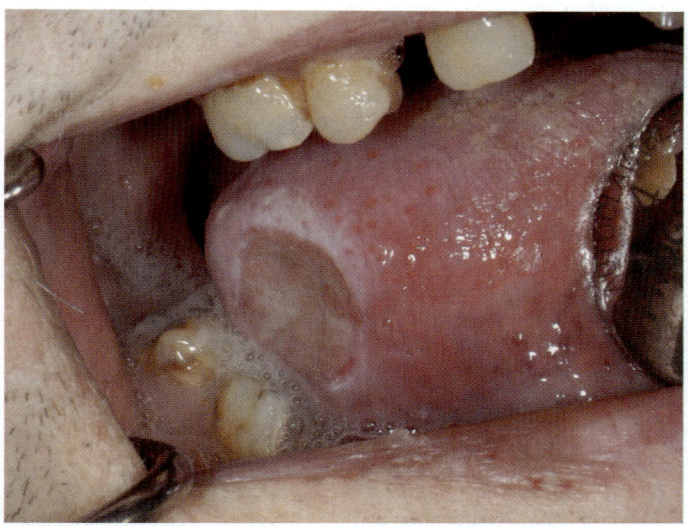

Photo 5. Longstanding traumatic ulcer of the right posterior lateral margin of the tongue

Table 10. Causes of mouth ulceration

Common causes	Less common causes

• trauma
  – from eating rough sharp foods
  – from sharp broken teeth, dental fillings, or dental appliances
• recurrent aphthous stomatitis
	• herpes simplex virus (primary herpetic gingivostomatitis, recurrent herpes stomatitis)
	• coxsackie viruses (herpangina, and hand, foot and mouth disease)
	• malignancies
	• drugs (as in erythema multiforme / Stevens-Johnson syndrome)
	• dermatoses (particularly lichen planus, mucous membrane pemphigoid, and pemphigus vulgaris)
	• systemic diseases (particularly Crohn's disease)

Aphthous ulcers

Recurrent aphthous stomatitis is the most common nontraumatic lesion of the oral mucosa. It is characterised by the periodic eruption of painful solitary or multiple ulcerations of the oral mucosa. The prevalence of recurrent aphthous stomatitis is between 5% and 25% in the general population; its onset is usually during childhood (with peak onset between 10 and 19 years), and the eruptions tend to diminish in frequency and severity with age. It generally occurs on the non-attached mucosa (eg of the cheek, lip and the floor of the mouth), rather than the gingivae and hard palate. Three forms are recognised:

- **Minor aphthous ulceration** is the most common form, presenting with ulcers that are 2 to 4 mm in diameter, occurring a few at a time and healing within 7 to 10 days.
- **Major aphthous ulceration**, a less common form, produces larger lesions of 10 mm or more that can persist for up to 6 weeks (and occasionally months) and heal with scarring.
- **Herpetiform aphthous ulceration** presents as recurrent crops of nonvesicular small ulcers, 1 to 2 mm in diameter, that coalesce to form larger ulcers, which heal within 1 to 2 weeks. Herpetiform aphthous ulcers are *not* caused by the herpes virus.

Assessment of aphthous stomatitis involves the exclusion of underlying causes by history, examination and, when required, relevant blood tests. Minor trauma (eg from toothbrushing or orthodontic appliances) may be a trigger for aphthous ulcers. They can be associated with deficiencies (eg iron, folate, vitamin B_{12}) and they often occur with coeliac or inflammatory bowel disease. Vitamin deficiency should be considered and, if suspected, blood tests should be performed, rather than vitamin supplements being given empirically. Aphthous ulcers can occur acutely with the cessation of smoking; in this situation they usually resolve with time. Behçet's syndrome is a rare condition featuring the association of oral aphthous ulceration with genital ulceration, eye disease and a wide variety of other systemic and cutaneous features.

Management

As a predominant trigger of aphthous ulcers is minor trauma, management of minor trauma is important (eg by changing oral hygiene practices, smoothing sharp edges of teeth or restorations, adjusting prostheses, or placing wax on orthodontic appliances).

For patients with mild aphthous stomatitis, topical anaesthetic agents (eg lignocaine gel every 3 hours) may be effective for symptomatic relief.

Active treatment of lesions by the application of topical corticosteroid cream or ointment can produce rapid healing, particularly if it is applied in the prodromal phase. Use:

1. *triamcinolone acetonide 0.1% paste topically to the lesions, 3 times daily after meals*

   OR

2. *betamethasone dipropionate 0.05% ointment topically to the lesions, 3 times daily after meals*

   OR

3. *beclomethasone dipropionate 50 micrograms sprayed onto the lesions, 3 times daily after meals.*

Management of patients with major aphthous ulceration, and management of immunocompromised patients with severe ulceration require specialist consultation. Treatment options may include intralesional corticosteroid or systemic (oral) prednis(ol)one.

Viral ulcers and herpes gingivostomatitis

Viral causes of oral ulceration include herpes simplex virus (primary herpetic gingivostomatitis, and recurrent infection) and coxsackie viruses (herpangina, and hand, foot and mouth disease).

Herpes simplex virus infection can be diagnosed by direct immunofluorescence or viral culture. Intraoral recurrent herpes ulceration is very rare; it occurs on the attached mucosa (eg of the gingivae, hard palate), whereas aphthous ulcers usually occur on the non-attached mucosa.

Recurrent herpes labialis is a result of latent virus reactivation in the trigeminal ganglion. It usually occurs on the vermilion of the lip and is relatively common, affecting approximately 15% of the population. The lesions are usually preceded by pain, burning, tingling or itching for several hours and up to two days; this is the prodromal phase and corresponds to an endothelial capillary response to virus that has arrived at the site from the trigeminal ganglion via the supplying sensory axons. The lesions begin as macules, rapidly become papular, with vesicles appearing within 48 hours and scabs appearing within 3 to 4 days; healing occurs without scarring.

Management

Mild cases can be treated symptomatically with systemic analgesic and topical anaesthetic drugs (eg lignocaine gel every 3 hours). Chlorhexidine mouthwash may prevent secondary intraoral lesions and act as an adjunct to oral hygiene; use:

chlorhexidine 0.2% mouthwash*, 10 mL held in the mouth for 1 minute, 2 to 3 times daily while the ulcers are present.

Chlorhexidine mouthwash is also available in combination with benzydamine, a topical analgesic. Topical corticosteroids are contra-indicated as they prevent attachment of white blood cells to virally infected epithelial cells and prevent virus destruction as well as aiding local spread.

Aciclovir cream has been shown to be effective for herpes labialis if applied at the first sign of the lesion (preferably during the prodrome):

aciclovir cream 5%, topically, 5 times daily (ie every 4 hours while awake) for 5 days.

Idoxuridine 0.5% with lignocaine is available in a cream that can be applied to the lesion frequently in the early stages of infection although it has not been proven to be effective.

Patients with severe herpes simplex virus infections (particularly in primary and progressive infection and if there is difficulty eating or swallowing) generally require systemic antiviral therapy. (See *Therapeutic Guidelines: Antibiotic* for antiviral treatments.)

Patients with severe herpes simplex virus infections requiring intra-venous therapy require specialist consultation.

---

* *With prolonged use (more than a few days), chlorhexidine may cause a superficial discolouration of the teeth and fillings (see p.59 for more information).*

Mucous membrane pemphigoid and pemphigus vulgaris

Mucous membrane pemphigoid (see Photo 6) and, less commonly, pemphigus vulgaris are uncommon autoimmune vesiculobullous disorders that affect stratified squamous epithelium. They can present as large, painful and persistent erosions in the mouth. Their onset is usually in middle to old age; they are more common in women than men.

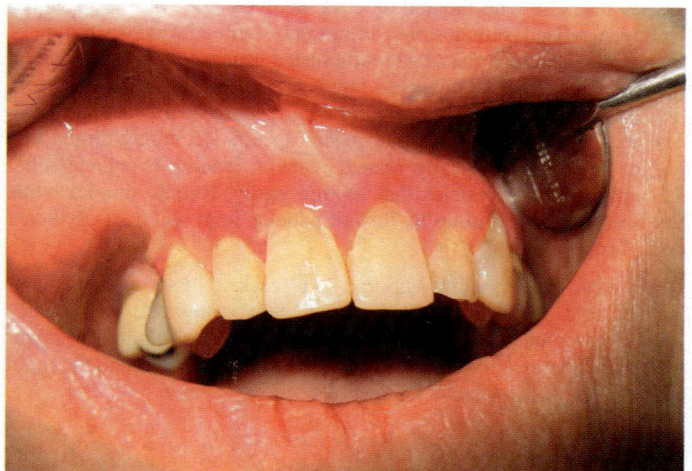

Photo 6. Mucous membrane pemphigoid manifesting as desquamative gingivitis

As their names suggest, mucous membrane pemphigoid is confined to the mucous membranes, whereas pemphigus vulgaris can affect all epithelial surfaces. In pemphigus vulgaris, the oral ulceration typically precedes the development of cutaneous lesions by six or more months.

Mucous membrane pemphigoid is characterised by subepithelial splitting, with bullae or vesicle formation occurring predominantly on the gingivae and palate. These heal with variable amounts of scar formation. The intraoral bullae of pemphigus vulgaris are intraepithelial and so are more fragile (than those of mucous membrane pemphigoid); they rupture easily, leaving large erosive mucosal lesions.

Diagnosis and treatment require specialist consultation and management. Definitive diagnosis requires a biopsy of tissue, and is based on histological features as well as immunofluorescence studies of fresh tissue. Biopsy of the markedly fragile tissues of pemphigoid and pemphigus requires a high level of skill.

Management is often protracted and usually requires oral immunosuppressive therapy with corticosteroids, azathioprine or cyclosporin, alone, or in combination with a topical immunosuppressant.

Erythema multiforme

Erythema multiforme is an acute and sometimes recurrent hypersensitivity reaction, with the oral mucosa involved alone or in association with generalised skin lesions. It presents with a wide spectrum of severity. It is characterised by blood-crusted lips, severe and widespread oral ulceration and, sometimes, target lesions on the skin. Erythema multiforme occurs mainly in young adults, more commonly in males. There is a wide variety of predisposing factors (including drugs) that trigger an immunologically related reaction leading to subepithelial and intraepithelial vesicles that rupture easily. Herpes simplex virus has been implicated in up to 70% of patients with recurrent erythema multiforme.

Healing can be very slow—up to 3 to 6 weeks. No specific treatment is available, but supportive care is very important with early ophthalmological and dermatological specialist consultation. Urgent referral of all cases for specialist assessment is advised due to the rapid onset of severe sequelae in many cases.

FUNGAL INFECTIONS

Oral candidosis

Oral candidosis (oral candidiasis) has many clinical presentations. Oral candidosis is uncommon in healthy individuals. It is always an opportunistic infection with predisposing factors that may be either local or systemic (see Table 11). Oral candidosis is extremely uncommon in healthy individuals.

Oral candidosis can usually be diagnosed on clinical appearance, although microscopy of a smear specimen and culturing of saliva can be helpful.

The creamy white plaques of thrush (pseudomembranous candidosis), which are not fixed to the oral mucosa, are easily recognisable. Once removed, these plaques leave red inflamed mucosa. Some plaques remain tenacious and can only be removed with difficulty and some discomfort. Other forms of candidosis, such as acute erythematous

Table 11. Predisposing factors in oral candidosis

Local factors	Systemic factors
• the wearing of dentures • xerostomia	• immunosuppression (eg human immunodeficiency virus, leukaemia) • endocrine disturbances • the use of some medications (eg inhaled and systemic corticosteroids, antibiotics)

candidosis (eg tender red mucosa after antibiotics) and chronic erythematous candidosis (eg red inflamed mucosa that is in contact with the fitting surface of dentures), are often misdiagnosed.

Hyperplastic candidosis presents as a fixed lesion on the oral mucosa; it is usually white. It can sometimes clinically resemble oral cancer; therefore biopsy is important to confirm the diagnosis. The clinician must remain aware that this condition frequently has an associated dysplasia and, irrespective of the initial histopathology report, the area must remain under review with early re-biopsy if resolution is not achieved.

Management

Exclude underlying predisposing factors, especially in recurrent cases of oral candidosis. Correct local precipitating factors, such as ill-fitting dentures, and address oral hygiene. At night, dentures should be removed, cleaned thoroughly, and twice weekly soaked in white vinegar (diluted approximately 1:20) or a 1% solution of sodium hypochlorite (common bleach).

Treat with:

1 *miconazole* 2% gel, 2.5 mL (child younger than 1 year: 1.25 mL) topically (then swallowed), 4 times daily, after meals, for 14 to 21 days (measuring spoon supplied with pack). Place directly in mouth and on tongue or, if dentures are present, place on the cleaned fitting surface immediately prior to insertion*

   OR

2 *amphotericin† 10 mg lozenge sucked, 4 times daily for 14 to 21 days*

   OR

---

* Miconazole can potentiate the effect of warfarin.

† Do not use amphotericin lozenges in patients with severe xerostomia, as the action of sucking lozenges can cause further trauma and irritation to the oral mucosa.

3. *nystatin 100 000 units/mL suspension, 1 mL topically (then swallowed), 6-hourly for 7 to 14 days.*

Advise denture wearers with oral candidosis to apply the antifungal agent to the cleaned fitting surface of the dentures before inserting them.

The management of severe disease in immunocompromised patients (eg those with HIV) requires specialist consultation. This may require the use of systemic antifungal drugs such as fluconazole or itraconazole. Long-term treatment may be required.

Angular cheilitis

Angular cheilitis presents as an erythematous skin plaque usually with formation of fissuring at one or both corners of the mouth, often associated with intraoral candidal infection. Other organisms implicated are staphylococci and streptococci. Facial skin folds and wrinkling at the corners of the mouth and along the nasolabial fold leads to a chronically moist environment that predisposes to angular cheilitis.

The angular fold becomes more pronounced in edentulous patients, especially if dentures are not worn. Saliva can accumulate in this fold, producing maceration and eventually cheilitis. New dentures can sometimes help correct this excessive folding, and therefore a dental review is recommended.

Other factors implicated in the causation of angular cheilitis are atopic and seborrhoeic dermatitis, iron deficiency anaemia and vitamin B_{12} or folate deficiency. Vitamin deficiency should be considered and, if suspected, blood tests should be performed, rather than vitamin supplements being given empirically. Diabetes has been implicated, but angular cheilitis and intraoral candidosis have not been shown to occur at increased frequency in patients with diabetes, irrespective of the level of control of their diabetes.

Microscopy of a swab specimen can aid in the diagnosis of angular cheilitis.

Treat oral candidosis if present (see p.119). In addition, use:

1. *miconazole* 2% cream or gel topically to the angles of the mouth, 4 times daily for at least 14 days*

   OR

1. *nystatin 100 000 units/g cream topically to the angles of the mouth, 2 to 3 times daily for at least 14 days.*

---

* *Miconazole can potentiate the effect of warfarin.*

Management of persistent angular cheilitis requires specialist consultation.

ORAL MUCOSITIS AND XEROSTOMIA

Oral mucositis

Oral mucositis refers to erythema and ulceration of the mucosal surfaces of the oral cavity due to cancer treatment modalities such as radiotherapy and/or chemotherapy. It is sometimes also referred to as stomatitis. Other causes of oral mucosal inflammation include xerostomia and nutritional causes (eg hypovitaminosis). In most instances, a history and careful examination clarifies the underlying cause.

Oral mucositis can lead to significant problems with eating, drinking and compliance with medications. In addition, patients undergoing cancer treatment who develop mucositis have an increased risk of systemic infection. They require longer hospital admissions and sometimes treatment modification or cessation because of their mucositis.

To reduce the morbidity associated with cancer treatment, patients should be dentally fit before commencing radiotherapy to the head and neck region or chemotherapy, particularly if the treatment regimen will result in severe mucositis and xerostomia. Dental treatment should be modified to suit the patient's need and circumstance, and should be performed in coordination with the patient's cancer treatments. Dental extraction sockets generally heal well in patients undergoing chemotherapy, whereas the chances of osteoradionecrosis can be very high in patients who have received radiotherapy. Caution is required when treating patients who have a history of taking bisphosphonates, and specialist advice should be sought. (See p.85 for osteoradionecrosis, and pp.76–9 for information about patients taking bisphosphonates.)

The patient should be warned of the probability of mucositis (and its nature and likely duration) before beginning treatment.

For further information on mucositis, see *Therapeutic Guidelines: Palliative Care*.

Management

Management of oral mucositis is essentially palliative, often requiring mouthwashes to reduce pain, relieve inflammation and allow some oral dietary intake. Patients with profound mucositis are unable to undertake normal oral hygiene, although this should be encouraged as much as is physically possible. There is currently no widely available treatment for oral mucositis. Preparations containing chlorhexidine are not recommended for the specific treatment of mucositis; however, they are useful in assisting to maintain oral hygiene in patients unable to adequately brush their teeth because of oral discomfort. A list of available medications is given in Table 12; however, there are conflicting data relating to their usefulness. A number of other drugs, including palifermin and amifostine, are under trial for severe oral mucositis secondary to chemotherapy and radiotherapy. These are currently restricted to use in cancer specialist centres.

Xerostomia

Xerostomia is a relatively common condition. Xerostomia refers to the subjective complaint of a dry mouth which may or may not occur in the context of reduced salivary flow. The objective dry mouth should, in fact, be referred to as 'salivary gland hypofunction'; however, common usage has resulted in the term 'xerostomia' being used for both subjective and objective dry mouth. For this reason, xerostomia is used throughout this text.

Xerostomia is due to salivary gland dysfunction and there may be a reduction in both the quantity and the quality of saliva. There are many physiological and pathological conditions that can result in xerostomia; these may be developmental, inflammatory or neoplastic.

Xerostomia most commonly occurs as an adverse effect of drugs; the most frequently implicated drugs are tricyclic antidepressants, antihistamines and anticholinergics. Patients should be warned if xerostomia is a possible adverse effect of any drug they are prescribed. This is particularly important for patients with chronic conditions, who may be taking medications for a long time. Xerostomia is also a common adverse effect of some recreational drugs (eg marijuana, heroin) and is implicated in the profound deterioration of the teeth that is observed in people with drug dependencies. Injecting drug users have a higher prevalence of hepatitis C infection than the general community, and a common extrahepatic manifestation of hepatitis C infection is xerostomia.

Long-term drug use results in prolonged xerostomia that can have a profound effect on the teeth. This not only causes a marked increase in the rate of caries, but also causes significant worsening of any periodontal disease. The end result of this long-term xerostomia is dental pain (which is occasionally masked by the drugs) and loss of teeth. Prevention of these dental diseases is possible, but only if preventive measures are instituted early.

Table 12. Oral preparations available for mucositis and xerostomia

Agent	Method of use	Purpose
Antiplaque/antibacterial preparations		
chlorhexidine 0.2% mouthwash alcohol-free	dilute 5 mL mouthwash with 5 mL water, rinse twice daily	may assist with cleansing of mucositis and shifting of mucous plaques on mucosal surfaces oral hygiene adjunct
chlorhexidine 0.12% mouthwash alcohol-free	use without dilution; rinse with 5 mL twice daily	can be used by people having concurrent chemotherapy and by people with chemotherapy-induced mucositis limits exposure to water-borne pathogens oral hygiene adjunct may assist with cleansing of mucositis and shifting of mucous plaques on mucosal surfaces
chlorhexidine 0.12% gel alcohol-free	apply when needed to all mucosal surfaces and gingival margins	oral hygiene adjunct provides lubrication eases discomfort
Anti-inflammatory and pain-relief preparations		
benzydamine hydrochloride 0.15% solution	rinse 10–15 mL, 4 to 6 times daily (not to be swallowed)	provides some pain relief
Lubrication preparations		
lip balm with chlorhexidine	apply as necessary	useful for lip mucositis
artificial saliva	apply as necessary	transient relief of oral dryness

Salivary gland agenesis is a congenital anomaly that can cause profound xerostomia in children. Xerostomia can be associated with connective tissue disorders that result in either primary or secondary Sjögren's syndrome, which occurs predominantly in postmenopausal women. Xerostomia may also be a direct effect of head and neck radiotherapy, with the degree of salivary flow reduction being dependent on the dose and region of the radiation.

A decrease in the quantity and/or the quality of saliva has a profound effect on the oral environment resulting in extensive and recurrent smooth surface dental decay, increased periodontal disease, significant worsening of any underlying mucosal disease, increased likelihood of oral candidosis and significant difficulty with the retention of dentures. There may also be difficulty with mastication, swallowing and speech.

For further information on xerostomia, see *Therapeutic Guidelines: Palliative Care*.

Management

Ideally, before patients commence taking medications that can cause xerostomia, they should have a detailed dental check-up followed by treatment of any active disease. Topical fluoride can be used to reduce demineralisation and to promote remineralisation. Other topical agents such as tooth cream may also be used to promote remineralisation of the teeth. (See Table 9, p.95, for topical applications used for caries reduction.) Anecdotal reports from patients indicate that this also diminishes the feeling of oral dryness that so profoundly affects their quality of life. The patient should be given oral hygiene instruction, and review appointments should be at 4- to 6-monthly intervals.

Artificial saliva can be considered, but the effects are often too transient to be of significant benefit. A range of products (eg throat lozenges and chewing gum) that stimulate salivary flow may give temporary relief from oral dryness in some patients. However, many of these products either are very acidic or have high sugar content and can further increase demineralisation of teeth. A further complication of xerostomia is that extractions may leave the patient unable to cope with dentures. Thus, good oral hygiene, regular dental examinations and treatments as necessary, and topical remineralisation agents are of paramount importance in patients with long-term xerostomia.

Oral preparations that are used for mucositis (see Table 12, p.123) may be useful in the symptomatic management of xerostomia. The use of systemic secretogogues for salivary stimulation has been assessed, with mixed results. Pilocarpine is probably the most widely studied of these agents; it is a parasympathomimetic drug, functioning as a muscarinic cholinergic agonist. Research is varied as to its usefulness; its effects are relatively short-lived, and in some patients it has profound adverse effects. Recent studies indicate that it may be suitable as a topical agent; however, further evidence is required before this can be recommended.

FURTHER READING

eTG complete [CD-ROM]. Melbourne: Therapeutic Guidelines Limited [regularly updated].

Medications in dentistry supplement. Aust Dent J 2005;50(4 Suppl 2): S1–81.

Acute odontogenic infections

Acute odontogenic (or tooth-related) infections are common. They arise from either the dental pulp (secondary to restoration breakdown, caries, or loss of tooth structure from trauma), the periodontal tissues (most commonly the result of advanced periodontitis), or the pericoronal tissues (most commonly from partially impacted mandibular third molars). The infection usually consists of mixed anaerobic and aerobic oral bacteria. The process of odontogenic infection always commences in the vicinity of the tooth. If ignored or inappropriately treated, it progresses to a localised abscess, then spreads beyond the confines of the jaws to the facial or neck soft tissues. Occasionally it becomes Ludwig's angina or spreads to the brain or mediastinum. The medical status of the patient is very important, particularly if the patient is immunocompromised.

An acute odontogenic infection should be considered as an emergency, and management should be commenced preferably within 24 hours. The first line of management should be by appropriate dental procedure, with medications sometimes used as adjunctive therapy. If patients seek advice from medical practitioners, they should be promptly directed to a dental practitioner. However, patients often seek (or are given) antibiotic-only treatment, obtain initial symptomatic relief, and then avoid seeking dental treatment. This is potentially serious and may lead to severe odontogenic infections.

LOCALISED DENTAL INFECTION

The various types of odontogenic infections are presented in Figure 2 (p.128). A localised dental abscess is a collection of pus that can be periapical, pericoronal or periodontal in origin.

Treatment of localised odontogenic infections

Odontogenic infections require clinical dental management to remove the source of the infection. This can be by extraction, endodontic (root canal) treatment, or periodontal treatment (see Box 11, p.128).

Antibiotics should be considered *only* when the infection has spread beyond the confines of the jaw and has produced facial swelling, or

continued on p.129

Figure 2. Schematic diagram of some odontogenic infections and the stages of dental caries (decay)

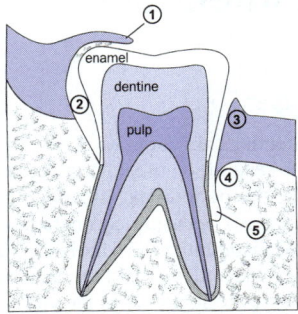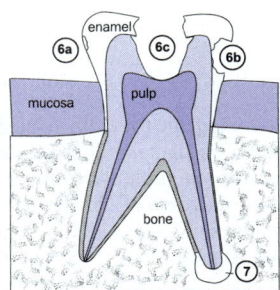

Diagram showing pericoronal disease and periodontal disease on the left tooth, and caries and its sequelae on the right tooth:

1. Pericoronal infection
2. Pericoronal abscess
3. Gingivitis
4. Periodontitis (bone loss)
5. Periodontal abscess
6. Caries
   a. 'white spot'
   b. initial cavity
   c. large cavity involving the pulp
7. Periapical lesion or abscess

Box 11. Treatment options for localised acute odontogenic infections

Periapical abscess
- Endodontic (root canal) treatment
- Extraction

Periodontal abscess
- Periodontal treatment (scaling, root planing)
- Extraction

Pericoronal infection
- Local treatment
  - Remove or recontour the opposing tooth if it is impinging on the operculum
  - Irrigate with sterile solution
  - Warm saline or chlorhexidine mouthwashes
- Extraction

when there are systemic symptoms and fever. Antibiotic use is then an *adjunct* to physical dental treatment (not a replacement). Antibiotics should *not* be used for dental pain, pulpitis, or infection localised to the teeth, nor to cover delay in providing dental treatment.

SPREADING DENTAL INFECTIONS

The consequence of untreated localised dental disease is that it may spread into the surrounding tissues. Spreading dental infections may be superficial (involving the canine or buccal spaces) or deep (involving the upper neck). The treatment of spreading dental infection—regardless of whether an abscess (a collection of pus) or cellulitis (an infected inflammatory swelling)—is by removal of the cause, via endodontic or periodontal treatment or extraction, and drainage of any pus.

General principles for the management of infection are:
- remove the cause
- drain the pus
- support the patient with analgesia and rehydration
- consider antibiotics.

Superficial infections

Most superficial infections can be treated with local surgical or dental treatment alone.

In patients who have **severe superficial infections** with swelling and systemic signs and symptoms, antibiotic therapy should be used in addition to local surgical or dental treatment:

1 *phenoxymethylpenicillin 500 mg (child: 10 mg/kg up to 500 mg) orally, 6-hourly for 5 days*

   OR

2 *amoxycillin 500 mg (child: 10 mg/kg up to 500 mg) orally, 8-hourly for 5 days*

   OR (for patients hypersensitive to penicillins)

3 *clindamycin 300 mg (child: 7.5 mg/kg up to 300 mg) orally, 8-hourly for 5 days.*

Children hypersensitive to penicillins who are unable to take capsules (the only oral formulation of clindamycin available in Australia) require specialist input for their management.

For **unresponsive infections**, use:

1. *metronidazole 400 mg (child: 10 mg/kg up to 400 mg) orally, 12-hourly for 5 days*

    PLUS

    1. *phenoxymethylpenicillin 500 mg (child: 10 mg/kg up to 500 mg) orally, 6-hourly for 5 days*

        OR

    2. *amoxycillin 500 mg (child: 10 mg/kg up to 500 mg) orally, 8-hourly for 5 days*

    OR

2. *amoxycillin+clavulanate 875+125 mg (child: 22.5+3.2 mg/kg up to 875+125 mg) orally, 12-hourly for 5 days*

    OR (for patients hypersensitive to penicillins)

3. *clindamycin 300 mg (child: 7.5 mg/kg up to 300 mg) orally, 8-hourly for 5 days.*

Children hypersensitive to penicillins who are unable to take capsules (the only oral formulation of clindamycin available in Australia) require specialist input to their management.

If superficial infections are inadequately treated, they may spread—canine fossa infections may spread intracranially via the orbital veins; buccal space infections may spread to the neck and become deep infections. Both can lead to life-threatening situations.

> ***All patients with infection should be reviewed within 48 to 72 hours of commencing treatment.***

The patient should be advised that if their condition deteriorates, they should contact the dental practitioner and be reviewed promptly. If the infection has not resolved within five days, *do not* just 'repeat the antibiotic'. Check that the cause has been removed, any pus has been drained, the appropriate antibiotic is being used for the particular microbial sensitivity, and the patient's general condition and medical situation are being managed.

Deep infections

Odontogenic infections that spread to the submandibular and pharyngeal spaces in the upper neck are potentially life-threatening, as there is a risk of airway obstruction. Any patient who has trismus and cannot open their mouth more than 2 cm (interincisal) must be assessed for signs of airway compromise. Signs and symptoms of airway compromise include stridor (noisy breathing), dyspnoea (difficult breathing), dysphagia (difficulty in swallowing), and elevation and firmness of the tongue.

Patients with deep infections and a compromised airway must be assessed urgently by an oral and maxillofacial surgeon or other surgical or anaesthetic specialist with training in the management of such patients.

> ***Patients with trismus and breathing or swallowing difficulty require urgent referral to an appropriate specialist or hospital emergency department (they should not be sent away with antibiotics for review later).***

Patients with systemic symptoms of pain and dehydration usually need to be managed in hospital, particularly if the infection is extensive. Management involves removal of the tooth, drainage, microbial culture and sensitivities of causative organisms, and treatment with intravenous antibiotics. For empirical treatment, use:

metronidazole 500 mg (child: 12.5 mg/kg up to 500 mg) IV, 12-hourly

PLUS

1. *benzylpenicillin 1.2 g (child: 30 mg/kg up to 1.2 g) IV, 6-hourly*

   OR

2. *amoxy/ampicillin 2 g (child: 50 mg/kg up to 2 g) IV, 6-hourly*

   OR (for patients hypersensitive to penicillins, excluding immediate hypersensitivity)

2. *cephazolin 1 g (child: 25 mg/kg up to 1 g) IV, 8-hourly*

   OR (for patients with immediate hypersensitivity to penicillins)

3. *clindamycin 450 mg (child: 10 mg/kg up to 450 mg) IV, 8-hourly*

   OR

3. *lincomycin 600 mg (child: 15 mg/kg up to 600 mg) IV, 8-hourly.*

Continue the intravenous regimen until the drains cease being productive, or swelling and trismus cease (and the patient can swallow), then change to an oral regimen (see p.130) for a further five days.

Ludwig's angina

Classically, Ludwig's angina is a severe bilateral cellulitis involving all of the neck spaces from the mandible to the thoracic inlet. Patients with Ludwig's angina are severely ill, and have a significant risk of death. If death occurs, it is usually from airway obstruction. (Angina means 'strangling', so the condition is well named.) Older medically compromised patients may die of multiorgan failure secondary to septicaemia.

It has become common to call all severe deep neck infections 'Ludwig's angina', which is technically incorrect. However, inadequately treated deep neck infections can progress to Ludwig's angina. The treatment is as for deep infection (see pp.130–1).

Patients with Ludwig's angina require urgent referral to an appropriate specialist or hospital emergency department.

POST–DENTOALVEOLAR SURGERY INFECTION

Post–dentoalveolar surgery infection is uncommon (3% to 5%) and is of similar incidence regardless of whether prophylactic antibiotics have been given or not. It is often confused with postsurgical inflammation, or dry socket (see p.134). The specific signs of dentoalveolar surgical infection are:

- cellulitis (ie a hot tense swelling)
- fluctuation
- purulent discharge from the extraction or surgical site for more than 72 hours after surgery
- pain and swelling that either worsens or fails to improve 48 hours after surgery
- persistent hyperpyrexia (more than 39 °C at 48 hours or more after surgery).

Laboratory markers can also be used to identify evidence of infection.

A radiograph to exclude the presence of residual roots or bony sequestra should be taken.

Management

Management must include drainage of any pus collection. Hourly wound irrigation (with, for example, warm saline or chlorhexidine 0.2%) is helpful.

If there are systemic signs or the patient is medically compromised, consider using antibiotics:

1. *phenoxymethylpenicillin 500 mg (child: 10 mg/kg up to 500 mg) orally, 6-hourly for 5 days*

   OR

2. *amoxycillin 500 mg (child: 10 mg/kg up to 500 mg) orally, 8-hourly for 5 days*

   OR (for patients hypersensitive to penicillins)

3. *clindamycin 300 mg (child: 7.5 mg/kg up to 300 mg) orally, 8-hourly for 5 days.*

In more severe or unresponsive cases, use:

1. *metronidazole 400 mg (child: 10 mg/kg up to 400 mg) orally, 12-hourly for 5 days*

   PLUS

   1. *phenoxymethylpenicillin 500 mg (child: 10 mg/kg up to 500 mg) orally, 6-hourly for 5 days*

      OR

   2. *amoxycillin 500 mg (child: 10 mg/kg up to 500 mg) orally, 8-hourly for 5 days*

   OR (for patients hypersensitive to penicillins)

   2. *clindamycin 300 mg (child: 7.5 mg/kg up to 300 mg) orally, 8-hourly for 5 days.*

For pain, use paracetamol or a nonsteroidal anti-inflammatory drug. See pp.145–55 for discussion of management of post-treatment pain.

For patients who require intravenous antibiotics, specialist consultation should be sought (see p.131 for intravenous regimens).

Severe postsurgical infections that have spread beyond the confines of the jaws are clinically similar to spreading infections and should be managed similarly. See pp.129–32 for management of spreading infection.

Alveolar osteitis (dry socket)

Alveolar osteitis (localised osteitis, dry socket) presents as postoperative pain in and around an extraction socket that increases in severity between 1 and 3 days after the extraction. It is a common (approximately 5%) complication of tooth extraction. It is accompanied by a partially or totally disintegrated blood clot within the socket, with or without halitosis.

Alveolar osteitis is a failure of healing; however, it is commonly misdiagnosed as an infection. Alveolar osteitis should heal spontaneously in 2 to 3 weeks; however, it is recommended that the patient returns to a dental practitioner for treatment of the socket (with obtundent dressings), and other symptomatic measures, including analgesics and mouthwashes. Treatment with antibiotics once dry socket has developed is of no benefit.

If the pain persists for more than three weeks, or if there are signs beyond the socket, the diagnosis needs to be reviewed. Differential diagnoses include osteomyelitis, bisphosphonate-related osteonecrosis (see pp.76–9), and alveolar squamous cell carcinoma.

Antibiotic prophylaxis

Antibiotic prophylaxis is the prescription of antibiotics to minimise the risk of bacterial infection. It is given when the risk of infection is high. Infection can be at:
- a distant site, usually the heart (eg endocarditis)
- around an implanted foreign body (eg a joint prosthesis)
- at an oral surgical site (eg a dentoalveolar procedure).

PREVENTION OF ENDOCARDITIS

Prophylaxis for endocarditis is an accepted but unproven practice. There are no placebo-controlled trials demonstrating the efficacy of prophylactic antimicrobials, and population-based control studies have cast considerable doubt on the value of the practice. The evidence for effectiveness is based on animal models of endocarditis, and empirical observation. There is little or no cost benefit in treating patients with low-risk abnormalities having procedures with a low incidence of bacteraemia, and there is the added problem of morbidity due to adverse drug reactions.

Traditionally, the presence of 'significant bleeding' associated with a dental procedure has been taken as an indication for prophylaxis; however, bleeding has been shown to be a poor indicator of bacteraemia from dental procedures. Most dental procedures (excluding dental extractions and root planing) result in a bacteraemia no different from that occurring during hard chewing and toothbrushing. However, dental extractions (particularly in the presence of periodontal disease) and root planing *do* result in a substantial bacteraemia. See Figure 3 (p.139) for schematic representation of bacteraemia and dental procedures.

The following recommendations are based on current international practice. Discussion of the relative risks with the patient is advisable. The risks are different depending on the cardiac condition (see Table 13, p.136) and the dental procedure (see Table 14, p.137). Patients with high- or medium-risk cardiac conditions should be informed about dental preventive measures and should be helped to improve their oral and dental hygiene. Dental examination twice yearly is recommended.

Table 13. Cardiac conditions that have a risk for infective endocarditis with dental procedures

High-risk conditions	Medium-risk conditions	Low-risk conditions

• prosthetic cardiac valves
  – bioprosthetic
  – homograft
• previous infective endocarditis
• complex cyanotic congenital heart disease (transposition, tetralogy of Fallot)
• surgically constructed systemic-pulmonary shunts, or conduits
• mitral valve prolapse with clinically significant regurgitation
• acquired valvular dysfunction (eg rheumatic heart disease) in Indigenous patients
	• acquired valvular dysfunction (eg rheumatic heart disease) in non-Indigenous patients
	• congenital cardiac malformations other than those defined as high- or low-risk
	• hypertrophic cardiomyopathy
	• significant valvular/haemodynamic dysfunction associated with septal defects
		• isolated secundum atrial septal defects
		• surgical repair of septal defects
		• previous coronary artery bypass grafts or stents
		• mitral valve prolapse without regurgitation
		• physiological, functional or innocent murmur
		• previous Kawasaki disease without valvular dysfunction
		• cardiac pacemakers
		• pulmonary stenosis
		• heart-lung transplants

Patients with diabetes or renal impairment are at greater risk. Patients should be told to seek urgent medical attention if they detect possible symptoms of endocarditis (eg unexplained fever) following dental treatment.

The cardiac risk should be based on a thorough medical and imaging evaluation of the patient's current cardiac state. (In a recent Australian study*, 70% of patients who had been medically advised that they had a heart condition requiring antibiotic prophylaxis had a normal heart, and only 15% had a cardiac condition that requires antibiotic prophylaxis for dental extractions or root planing.)

Figure 3 (p.139) is a conceptual figure showing the relationship of dental procedure to bacteraemia and the threshold for antibiotic prophylaxis.

Table 15 (p.138) helps in making the decision about whether a patient with a cardiac condition requires antibiotic prophylaxis. Individual decisions need to be made about the risk versus the benefit of antibiotic prophylaxis for infective endocarditis (eg the benefits of prophylaxis

---

* Ching M, Straznicky I, Goss AN. *Cardiac murmurs: echocardiography in the assessment of patients requiring antibiotic prophylaxis for dental treatment. Aust Dent J 2005;50(4 Suppl 2):S69-73.*

Table 14. Dental procedures and their risk of causing a bacteraemia

High-risk procedures	Medium-risk procedures	Low-risk procedures
• extraction • periodontal procedures including surgery and root planing • replanting avulsed teeth • other surgical procedures (eg implant placement, apicoectomy)	• periodontal probing • intraligamentary and intraosseous local anaesthetic injection • supragingival calculus removal/cleaning • rubber dam placement with clamps (where risk of damaging gingiva) • restorative matrix band/strip placement • endodontics beyond the apical foramen • placement of orthodontic bands • placement of interdental wedges • subgingival placement of retraction cords, antibiotic fibres or antibiotic strips	• oral examination • infiltration and block local anaesthetic injection • restorative dentistry • supragingival rubber dam clamping and placement of rubber dam • intracanal endodontic procedures • removal of sutures • impressions and construction of dentures • orthodontic bracket placement and adjustment of fixed appliances • application of gels • intraoral radiographs • supragingival plaque removal

are more likely to outweigh the harms if a patient with a medium-risk cardiac condition is having a high-risk dental procedure rather than a medium-risk procedure). Key risk factors are the state of periodontal health and the nature and duration of the dental procedure.

If after careful evaluation of both the cardiac condition and the dental procedure (see Table 13 and Table 14) antibiotic prophylaxis is considered necessary (using Table 15, p.138), a single dose of antibiotic should be given before the procedure; there is no proven value to giving a follow-up dose six hours later. For standard prophylaxis use:

amoxycillin 2 g (child: 50 mg/kg up to 2 g) orally, 1 hour before the procedure
or amoxy/ampicillin 2 g (child: 50 mg/kg up to 2 g) IV, just before the procedure
or amoxy/ampicillin 2 g (child: 50 mg/kg up to 2 g) IM, 30 minutes before the procedure.

Table 15. Need for antibiotic prophylaxis for patients with a cardiac condition undergoing a dental procedure*

Cardiac condition \ Procedure	High-risk	Medium-risk	Low-risk
High-risk	YES	PROBABLE, but requirement for prophylaxis must be determined for each individual*	NO
Medium-risk	PROBABLE, but requirement for prophylaxis must be determined for each individual*	POSSIBLE, but requirement for prophylaxis must be determined for each individual*	NO
Low-risk	NO	NO	NO

* Individual decisions need to be made about the risk versus the benefit of antibiotic prophylaxis for infective endocarditis (eg a patient with a medium-risk cardiac condition having a high-risk dental procedure would be more closely considered for antibiotic prophylaxis than if they were having a medium-risk procedure). Key risk factors are the state of periodontal health and the nature and duration of the procedure.

Patients hypersensitive to penicillins, and those on long-term penicillin therapy or who have taken penicillin or a related beta-lactam antibiotic more than once in the previous month can use:

1 *clindamycin 600 mg (child: 15 mg/kg up to 600 mg) orally, 1 hour before the procedure*
or clindamycin 600 mg (child: 15 mg/kg up to 600 mg) IV over at least 20 minutes, just before the procedure

OR

1 *lincomycin 600 mg (child: 15 mg/kg up to 600 mg) IV over at least 1 hour, just before the procedure*

OR

2 *vancomycin 25 mg/kg up to 1.5 g (child younger than 12 years: 30 mg/kg up to 1.5 g) IV by slow infusion (over at least 60 minutes; rate not exceeding 10 mg/min), ending the infusion just before the procedure*

OR

3. *teicoplanin 400 mg (child: 10 mg/kg up to 400 mg) IV, just before the procedure*
   or teicoplanin 400 mg (child: 10 mg/kg up to 400 mg) IM, 30 minutes before the procedure.

There is no oral liquid formulation of clindamycin in Australia. An alternative for patients who are hypersensitive to penicillins (excluding immediate hypersensitivity), but *not* for those who have been on long-term penicillin or have taken a related beta-lactam antibiotic more than once in the previous month, is:

cephalexin 2 g (child: 50 mg/kg up to 2 g) orally, 1 hour before the procedure.

Figure 3. Conceptual figure showing the relationship of dental procedure to bacteraemia and the threshold for antibiotic prophylaxis*

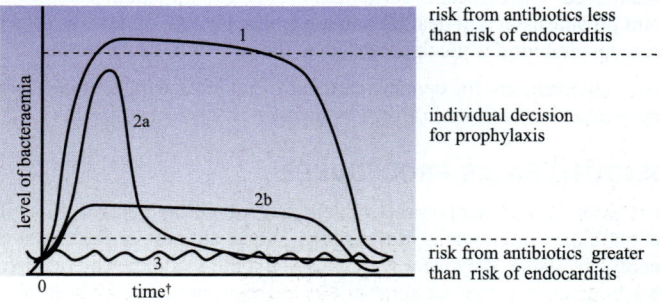

1. high-risk dental procedures—high prolonged bacteraemia
2. medium-risk dental procedures:
   a. high but short bacteraemia (eg clamp or wedge for patient with moderate to severe periodontal disease)
   b. low but prolonged bacteraemia (eg orthodontic band in patient with moderate periodontal disease)
3. low-risk dental procedures—background bacteraemia no different from physiological activity (eg chewing, toothbrushing)

* this diagram takes no account of cardiac risk
† bacteraemia usually does not persist for longer than 30 minutes after the end of the procedure

There is a subgroup of patients with a well-documented history of rheumatic fever (common in Indigenous Australians) who receive continuous prophylaxis against *Streptococcus pyogenes* infection. Patients with rheumatic valvular heart disease who are on regular prophylaxis with penicillin have a greater chance of penicillin-resistant organisms; they should be offered an antibiotic other than penicillin (ie clindamycin, lincomycin, vancomycin, teicoplanin [see pp.138–9]) for prophylaxis before a dental procedure.

PREVENTION OF INFECTION IN JOINT PROSTHESES

Patients with a joint prosthesis have an exceedingly low risk of infection at the prosthetic site by the haematogenous route. Traditionally, orthopaedic surgeons have advised patients with artificial joint prostheses that they need antibiotic cover for dental treatment; however, even with dental procedures where substantial bacteraemia is produced (eg dental extractions [particularly in the presence of periodontal disease], root planing), the value of antibiotic prophylaxis has not been established. The evidence, particularly for an asymptomatic established joint prosthesis in a fit healthy patient, is that the risk of adverse effects from an antibiotic is much greater than the risk from bacteraemia.

Recommendations for dental treatment of patients with artificial joint replacement are set out in Box 12 (pp.142–3).

DENTOALVEOLAR PROCEDURES

It is essential that dental practitioners understand the general principle of antibiotic prophylaxis for surgery. When antibiotics first became readily available, they were widely used in both medicine and dentistry as a 'protective cover' for surgery. However, prophylactic antimicrobial therapy must be restricted to situations in which it has been shown to be effective. For most dentoalveolar procedures in fit immunocompetent patients, antibiotic prophylaxis is *not* required or recommended. The low risk of wound infection must be balanced against the risk of adverse effects of the antibiotic.

Most surgical prophylaxis should be commenced *just* before the procedure. A single dose is usually adequate for operations lasting less than 2 hours. The aim is to achieve high plasma and tissue levels at the time that contamination is most likely (ie during the procedure).

Antibiotic prophylaxis should be *considered* for:
- surgical removal of a bone-impacted tooth or periapical surgery in a patient with a history of recurrent infections (patients with

evidence of active infection in the area of planned surgery do not have a prophylactic indication but may have a therapeutic indication)

- immunocompromised patients.

If antibiotic prophylaxis is required, give:

1. *phenoxymethylpenicillin 2 g (child: 40 mg/kg up to 2 g) orally, 1 hour before the procedure*

    OR

2. *amoxycillin 2 g (child: 50 mg/kg up to 2 g) orally, 1 hour before the procedure*
    or amoxy/ampicillin 2 g (child: 50 mg/kg up to 2 g) IV, just before the procedure
    or amoxy/ampicillin 2 g (child: 50 mg/kg up to 2 g) IM, 30 minutes before the procedure

    OR

2. *benzylpenicillin 1.2 g (child: 30 mg/kg up to 1.2 g) IV, just before the procedure*

    OR (if patient is hypersensitive to penicillins)

3. *clindamycin 600 mg (child: 15 mg/kg up to 600 mg) orally, 1 hour before the procedure*
    or clindamycin 600 mg (child: 15 mg/kg up to 600 mg) IV over at least 20 minutes, just before the procedure

    OR

3. *lincomycin 600 mg (child: 15 mg/kg up to 600 mg) IV over at least 1 hour, just before the procedure.*

Tooth extraction

The incidence of wound infection following simple extractions is negligible. The incidence following the removal of bone-impacted wisdom teeth in fit healthy patients is low (3% to 5%). An infection is usually, but not always, confined to the socket and of such low incidence that, generally, antibiotic prophylaxis is not recommended or required. Alveolar osteitis or 'dry socket' is *not* a bacterial infection but a wound-healing problem, and therefore antibiotics are of no value. (See p.134 for 'Alveolar osteitis'.)

Box 12. Recommendations for dental treatment of patients with artificial joint replacement

Prior to placement of the first artificial joint
- Referral to a dental practitioner for a comprehensive dental examination including radiographs.
- Appropriate treatments as indicated to make the patient orally and dentally fit.
- Dentist, if requested, to give a written opinion that the patient is orally and dentally fit.
- Arrangements made for regular dental review.

Dental problem in the first 3 months following artificial joint placement
- *Infection with abscess formation*:
  - Urgent and aggressive treatment of the abscess. Remove the cause (exodontic, endodontic or periodontal treatment) under antibiotic prophylaxis (see pp.137–9) (no need for continued antibiotics). See also 'Acute odontogenic infections' (p.127).
- *Noninfective dental problem without pain*:
  - Defer nonemergency dental treatment until 3 to 6 months after prosthesis placement.
- *Pain*:
  - Provide emergency dental treatment for pain.
  - Antibiotics should be considered if a high- or medium-risk dental procedure is performed (see Table 14, p.137).

Dental problem more than 3 months after artificial joint placement for patients with a normally functioning artificial joint
- Dental treatment (including extraction and root planing)— no antibiotic prophylaxis required.
- Regular dental review desirable.

Dental treatment for patients with significant risk factors for artificial joint infection
- Regular dental reviews essential.
- *Immunocompromised patients* (including those with insulin-dependent diabetes or systemic rheumatoid arthritis, those taking immunosuppressive treatment for organ transplants or malignancy, and those taking systemic corticosteroids [eg patients with severe asthma, dermatological problems]):
  - Consultation with the patient's treating physician is recommended, and antibiotic prophylaxis should be *considered* for all high-risk dental procedures (see Table 14, p.137).

continued next page

> **Box 12. Recommendations for dental treatment of patients with artificial joint replacement (cont.)**
>
> - *Failing, particularly chronically inflamed, artificial joints*:
>   - Consultation with the patient's treating orthopaedic surgeon is recommended, and antibiotic prophylaxis should be *considered* for all high-risk dental procedures (see Table 14, p.137).
>   - Defer nonessential dental treatment until orthopaedic problem has resolved.
> - *History of infected artificial joints*:
>   - Routine nonsurgical dental treatment—no prophylaxis indicated.
>   - High-risk dental procedures (eg extractions, root planing) (see Table 14, p.137)—antibiotics *required* (see pp.137–9).
>
> **Established infection by oral organisms on an artificial joint**
> - Urgent referral to dental practitioner to determine and eliminate any oral cause.
> - Aggressive treatment by removal of the cause, extraction or endodontic treatment under antibiotic prophylaxis.

Implants

Dental implants involve the elective surgical placement of foreign bodies into the jaw. Strict attention to surgical asepsis and technique is essential. The incidence of wound infection is very low and mainly relates to technique issues.

Controlled studies for both mandibular third molar surgery, and placement of dental implants show little or no benefit from antibiotic prophylaxis and there is a risk of adverse effects from antibiotics.

FURTHER READING

eTG complete [CD-ROM]. Melbourne: Therapeutic Guidelines Limited [regularly updated].

Medications in dentistry supplement. Aust Dent J 2005;50(4 Suppl 2): S1–81.

Post-treatment pain management

Dental pain is largely inflammatory in origin; however, there can be various causes or reasons for the inflammation.

An accurate diagnosis of the presenting condition must be formulated and the appropriate active dental treatment provided before considering the use of any adjunctive drugs, because the dental treatment is the most predictable means of reducing a patient's level of pain. (See 'Principles of diagnosis and prescribing', p.1, for how to form an accurate diagnosis.)

> *Dental treatment is the most predictable means of reducing pain of dental origin.*

An accurate diagnosis also helps to determine what type of adjunctive drugs (if any) may be effective (eg pain caused by infection may require an antibiotic, pain from inflammation may require an anti-inflammatory drug). Sometimes analgesics may be more appropriate—either alone or in conjunction with other medications.

UNDERSTANDING PAIN

Pain is a subjective phenomenon that is very difficult to measure; it depends on the patient's perception of pain, their coping strategies, and their previous experiences with pain and pain relief. The patient's confidence in the clinician's ability to diagnose and manage their problem may also play a role.

Both the level and the type of pain need to be assessed before the drug regimen is established. The level of pain is usually described as being mild, moderate or severe; the type of pain can be classified as nociceptive, neuropathic or psychogenic.

Nociceptive pain arises from stimulation of superficial or deep tissue receptors (nociceptors) as a result of tissue injury or inflammation. This is the most common type of pain in the dental setting.

Neuropathic pain arises from a disturbance of neural pathways at any point from the afferent conducting system to receptive centres in the central nervous system. Neuropathic pain is not uncommon among dental patients, but its diagnosis can be difficult to establish.

Psychogenic disorders (including **somatoform** pain disorders) are syndromes in which the patient presents with symptoms that predominantly suggest an organic disorder, but the medical history, physical examination and investigations do not demonstrate any organic disease that could explain the symptoms. There is usually no objective evidence of organic disease. Alternatively, an organic disorder may be present, but the symptoms experienced are in excess of, or disproportionate to, those usually seen with that level of organic disorder. These disorders can occur in the dental setting, and need to be identified early; a clinician who suspects that a patient has one of these disorders should refer the patient for further assessment by a specialist, rather than initiate any drug therapy.

Pain can also be classified as either acute or chronic:
- **Acute pain** is nociceptive in origin and it is the most common pain problem managed by dental practitioners. Fortunately, acute pain of oral and dental origin is relatively straightforward to diagnose, provided the clinician follows the recommended diagnostic processes, performs a thorough examination and conducts the appropriate tests. Most acute pain conditions of oral origin resolve rapidly once the appropriate dental treatment has been started; however, some patients require adjunctive analgesic therapy in the first 24 to 48 hours (or perhaps for slightly longer for patients with very severe pain).
- **Chronic pain** may be nociceptive, neuropathic, psychogenic or somatic in origin and hence can be difficult to diagnose accurately as there may not be any obvious signs or symptoms. It can also be difficult, if not impossible, to manage with analgesics alone, and other more appropriate management (including co-analgesics and psychological interventions) is required. It is often far more difficult to resolve than acute pain. Dental procedural treatment is usually counterproductive and should be discontinued in chronic oral neuropathic pain. For further information on the management of chronic pain, see *Therapeutic Guidelines: Analgesic* or standard texts.

PRINCIPLES OF USE OF ANALGESICS

Many practitioners have traditionally prescribed analgesics on a 'take as required for pain' basis rather than as a 'course of medication'. The take-as-required-for-pain approach results in poor pain management because the blood levels of the drug fluctuate considerably from peak levels to zero, with the associated pain levels ranging from excellent or good pain control to having recurrent pain, depending on the timing of when the medications are taken. That is, a cycle between pain and pain relief occurs with the patient often suffering more than is necessary, and the overall condition taking longer to resolve. See Box 13 (p.152) for further information.

Ideally, analgesics should be taken as a course of medication, whereby the patient is advised to take the medication at regular intervals for a specified period of time so the blood levels of the drug are maintained above the threshold level for effective pain relief. The time interval at which the next dose should be taken depends on the pharmacokinetic properties of the drug being used (such as its elimination half-life [an indication of the time taken for the drug to be cleared from the bloodstream] and protein binding capacity [amount of free drug available for pain relief]), drug formulation (eg immediate-release or modified-release preparations) and possible drug interactions. Most analgesics need to be taken every 4 or 6 hours. Using analgesics as a course of medication (rather than 'as required for pain') generally means that a shorter course of treatment is required and the drug can be stopped sooner; this particularly applies if the drug has both analgesic and anti-inflammatory properties.

Analgesics should be used at the lowest effective dose possible, and for as short a period of time as possible, to minimise the development of adverse effects and to reduce the chance of drug interactions with any other medications being taken at the same time.

The 'third molar model' has been used in many studies to compare the postoperative pain levels and effectiveness of various analgesics. Information about the results of the studies are outlined in Box 14 (p.154). The recommendations on pp.149–50 are based on findings from these studies.

Use of analgesics in dentistry

Analgesics should be used only when the patient's pain cannot be removed, reduced or controlled adequately by the appropriate dental treatment and with drugs that are appropriate for the presenting condition. Most painful dental and oral problems that require pain relief are due to inflammation of one of the oral, dental or associated tissues. This inflammation may be a result of various factors (eg infection, trauma, an operative procedure). Hence, assessment of the cause of the pain is essential as it dictates management.

Analgesics do not have any therapeutic effect—they essentially act by blocking the pain sensation being experienced by the patient. Analgesics should be considered only as an adjunct to the appropriate treatment (which may include other medications). Often, the treatment and other medications are effective, and therefore analgesics are usually only indicated for very severe pain situations, and only for short periods of time.

> Examples:
>
> If pain is caused by infection, the infection should be managed by operative procedures and drainage, with antimicrobial drugs (antibiotics, antifungal drugs or antiviral drugs) if adjunctive drug therapy is deemed necessary. Analgesics are given only if the pain persists.
>
> If pain is caused by inflammation, the irritating factors should be removed and anti-inflammatory drugs used as an adjunct to help reduce the inflammation more rapidly and more predictably. Analgesics are given only if the pain persists.

When analgesics are definitely required, an appropriate regimen of drug use should be established for each patient. If the patient can use nonsteroidal anti-inflammatory drugs (NSAIDs), then drugs that have combined analgesic and anti-inflammatory actions can be given. The combined action is generally more effective, because there is some reduction of inflammation at the site of origin of the pain in addition to the analgesic effect. If NSAIDs are contraindicated, the choice is essentially limited to paracetamol.

Route of administration

Most patients attending a dental practice for the management of dental, oral or facial pain are able to use **oral** analgesic preparations in the form of tablets, capsules or liquids. However, there are several reasons why patients may not tolerate oral medications:

- They may have difficulty swallowing tablets (eg because of physical or psychological problems).
- They may have difficulty absorbing drugs (eg because of gastric irritation, ulcers).
- If they have been taking multiple medications (either prescribed or self-administered, or both) in an attempt to manage their pain, they may have developed gastrointestinal symptoms (eg gastric irritation, nausea, vomiting).
- If they have not been eating or sleeping well, their ability to cope with pain may be markedly compromised.
- If they have been vomiting, oral medications may not be adequately absorbed by the stomach and the drugs may not reach adequate blood levels to be effective.

Alternative routes of administration are **parenteral** (injection) and **rectal** (suppositories). Suppositories can be very effective and are easy to use (although patient compliance is often difficult); parenteral preparations necessitate regular visits to a dentist, doctor or other suitable person, or hospitalisation.

PAIN MANAGEMENT STRATEGIES

Effective pain management begins with an accurate diagnosis and an appropriate treatment plan using the principle of the '3 Ds'—**D**iagnosis, **D**ental treatment and then **D**rugs (see p.4).

If pain relief with analgesics and/or anti-inflammatory medication is required for post-treatment pain, five questions must be answered before prescribing medications:

- Is the pain nociceptive in origin? If not, further investigations and other management approaches are required.
- Is the pain mild, moderate or severe? This estimation includes the patient's perception of the pain, and the clinician's assessment of the severity of the problem causing the pain.
- Has the appropriate dental treatment been provided? If not, it should be arranged immediately.
- Can the patient use nonsteroidal anti-inflammatory drugs (NSAIDs) (eg aspirin, ibuprofen, naproxen, ketorolac, ketoprofen)? If not, use paracetamol, with or without codeine. Typical contraindications to the use of NSAIDs are asthma, peptic ulceration and drug interactions (see pp.29–32).
- Can the patient take the medications via the oral route? If not, consider suppositories or parenteral preparations (see p.148).

Post-treatment pain management in adults

The clinical situation will indicate whether analgesics are likely to be required to help a patient manage their pain or the expected pain following dental treatment. The management strategies to be used will depend on the degree of pain:

For **mild pain**, use:

1 *ibuprofen 400 mg orally, 4-hourly (to a maximum of 2400 mg/24 hours)*

   OR

2. *aspirin 600 to 900 mg orally, 4-hourly (to a maximum of 3600 mg/24 hours)*

   OR (if NSAIDs are contraindicated)

3. *paracetamol 500 to 1000 mg orally, 4-hourly (to a maximum of 4 g/24 hours).*

For **moderate pain**, use:

1. *ibuprofen 400 to 600 mg orally, every 4 hours (to a maximum of 2400 mg/24 hours)*

   PLUS

   paracetamol+codeine 1000+60 mg orally, every 4 hours (to a maximum paracetamol dose of 4 g/24 hours)

   OR (if NSAIDs are contraindicated)

2. *paracetamol+codeine 1000+60 mg orally, every 4 hours (to a maximum paracetamol dose of 4 g/24 hours).*

For **severe pain**, use:

1. *ibuprofen 400 to 600 mg orally, every 4 hours (to a maximum of 2400 mg/24 hours)*

   PLUS

   paracetamol+codeine 1000+60 mg orally, every 4 hours (to a maximum paracetamol dose of 4 g/24 hours)

   OR (if NSAIDs are contraindicated)

2. *paracetamol+codeine 1000+60 to 1500+90 mg orally, every 4 hours (to a maximum paracetamol dose of 4 g/24 hours).*

If patients need to take both ibuprofen and paracetamol+codeine, the analgesic effect can be enhanced if the drugs are taken alternately at 2-hourly intervals (with each drug being taken every 4 hours only). The paracetamol+codeine can usually be stopped after 24 hours (or even the morning after the treatment is performed), but ibuprofen is useful for its anti-inflammatory effect for a further 2 to 3 days until the pain has completely resolved (see Box 14, p.154, for detailed explanation). If the patient has severe persistent pain (for more than five days), review the diagnosis and consider specialist referral.

The addition of doxylamine to any of the above regimens can sometimes have additional benefit. Doxylamine is an antihistamine that acts as a 'calmative' (which helps the patient cope with the pain). The patient must be warned that doxylamine can cause drowsiness. Commercial preparations are available that combine 10 mg of doxylamine with paracetamol+codeine. Such a preparation can be used if the calmative action is required as part of the post-treatment management of pain. In this case, the dosage of tablets used is based on the amount of paracetamol and codeine required, while also being mindful of the presence of the doxylamine. The dosage of doxylamine should not exceed 10 mg orally, 4-hourly.

If the patient has severe persistent pain (for more than five days), review the diagnosis and consider specialist referral.

Post-treatment pain management in children

Pain management in children is usually much simpler than in adults because of the lack of psychological overlay that usually modifies adults' responses to pain. However, the parent's response to their child being in pain needs to be considered, as the parent must provide the medication.

The paediatric patient is no different from the adult patient in requiring an accurate diagnosis of the origin of the pain, and appropriate dental treatment of the dental condition. Common procedures in children that can cause post-treatment pain are dental restorations, simple extractions and surgical extractions.

To limit post-treatment discomfort, it is important that procedural pain control is adequate—using a local anaesthetic and relative analgesia (using, for example, an inhalational agent such as nitrous oxide), or a general anaesthetic to limit emotional overlay is the initial step in pain control.

Analgesia using simple drugs (ie paracetamol or a nonsteroidal anti-inflammatory drug [NSAID]) is generally the cornerstone of pain management in children. Aspirin should *not* be used in children because of the risk of Reye's syndrome.

For post-treatment pain in children, use:

1 *ibuprofen 5 to 10 mg/kg orally, 6- to 8-hourly (to a maximum daily dose of 2400 mg)*

   OR

1 *paracetamol 15 mg/kg orally or rectally, 4- to 6-hourly (to a maximum daily dose of 4 g).*

continued on p.153

Box 13. Combining the use of ibuprofen with paracetamol+codeine for enhanced pain management in adults

If ibuprofen is taken first, and immediately after the emergency dental treatment, it can provide effective pain relief as the local anaesthetic is wearing off. It will also begin its anti-inflammatory action (which will help to minimise pain, or prevent it entirely, by reducing the inflammatory action in the affected tissues). As the main action of ibuprofen is local (ie at the site of inflammation) and paracetamol and codeine work within the central nervous system, ibuprofen and paracetamol+codeine are complementary.

Figure 4 illustrates schematically how analgesia can be enhanced when ibuprofen and paracetamol+codeine are given alternately at 2-hourly intervals. After the initial lag time, the blood level of ibuprofen reaches a concentration above the threshold level for effective pain relief (point 'a'). After some time, its effective blood level falls below the threshold level and it becomes ineffective as an analgesic (point 'c'). However, if paracetamol+codeine is given 2 hours after the ibuprofen, the ibuprofen is still above its threshold level for effective analgesia while the paracetamol+codeine is being absorbed. The paracetamol+codeine will then reach its threshold level for pain relief (point 'b') approximately 30 minutes before the ibuprofen level falls below its effective threshold (point 'c').

Figure 4. Schematic representation of blood levels of drugs taken alternately for the management of severe pain

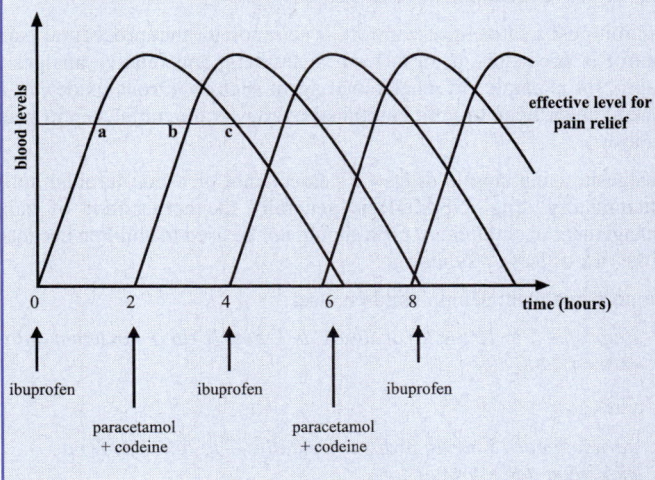

continued next page

> It is not essential to use the above drug regimen, and patients can still have effective pain relief if they take the ibuprofen and the paracetamol+codeine at the same time and then every 4 hours. However, there may be some fluctuation in pain levels towards the end of each 4-hour period and before full absorption 30 to 60 minutes after the next dose.
>
> The paracetamol+codeine can usually be stopped the next morning or after 24 hours, but the ibuprofen should be continued for a further 2 to 3 days since its anti-inflammatory effect will help with further resolution of the inflammation that caused the pain.
>
> The alternating regimen may reduce the gastric irritation effects as the stomach is not subjected to the three different drugs (ibuprofen, codeine, paracetamol) all at the same time.
>
> The alternating regimen relies on patient compliance (which requires that the patient understands the rationale for taking the drugs at different times). The patient can be provided with a written set of specific instructions outlining the times to take each drug (ie rather than telling the patient 'every 2 hours', specify the exact time [eg 2.30 pm]). A simple 'timeline' such as that shown in Figure 5 can be given to the patient with the times and drugs adjusted for the patient's particular needs.
>
> **Figure 5. Example of instructions for a patient following surgery (using a timeline)**
>
>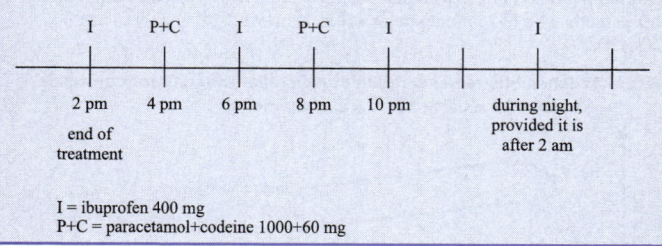
>
> I = ibuprofen 400 mg
> P+C = paracetamol+codeine 1000+60 mg

As the main action of ibuprofen is local (ie at the site of inflammation) and paracetamol and codeine work within the central nervous system, they are complementary, and so they can be combined.

It is important that post-treatment analgesics are given regularly and in adequate doses.

In some circumstances when post-treatment pain is severe, opiates such as codeine may be required in addition to the other agents. Nocturnal discomfort may be alleviated with nocturnal sedation using promethazine, which can be combined with paracetamol for effective pain relief.

If pain persists after 24 hours, the patient should be reassessed.

Box 14. How the recommendations for pain management were derived

The 'third molar model' has been used in many studies to compare the postoperative pain levels and effectiveness of various analgesics.

These studies have consistently shown that codeine alone is not very effective as an analgesic but its effectiveness increases when it is combined with paracetamol or aspirin. Increasing the dose of both the codeine and paracetamol increases the effectiveness of pain relief for this combination of drugs. However, ibuprofen has been shown to be an even better analgesic drug, particularly as the dose increases (see Figure 6).

Codeine can be prescribed alone or in combination with paracetamol (or other drugs). There are a variety of both 'over-the-counter' preparations (with lower doses of codeine) and prescription-only combinations of paracetamol+codeine.

At least 25 to 30 mg of codeine is required for effective analgesia, so combined preparations with a lower dose of codeine are usually inadequate. However, the compounds containing 30 mg codeine provide very effective analgesia, particularly if a double dose is taken (which is generally required for severe pain).

Combining doxylamine with paracetamol+codeine provides an alternative for patients who have moderate or severe pain who are unable to use NSAIDs.

Figure 6. Schematic representation of pain relief with different systemic medications using the 'third molar model'

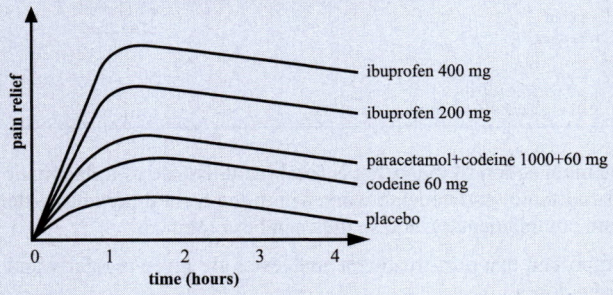

Figure 6 is a schematic diagram of the results of trials using the third molar model. All the drugs are effective for about 4 hours; however, there is a 'lag time' while each tablet is being absorbed, and then a 'tapering off' effect as the blood level drops after reaching its peak. There is wide variation between individual patients.

FURTHER READING

Dionne RA, Phero JC, Becker DE. Management of pain and anxiety in the dental office. Philadelphia: WB Saunders Co. 2002.

eTG complete [CD-ROM]. Melbourne: Therapeutic Guidelines Limited [regularly updated].

Hargreaves K, Keiser K, Byrne E. Analgesics in endodontics. In: Cohen S, Burns RC, editors. Pathways of the pulp. St Louis: Mosby; 2005.

Holstein A, Hargreaves KM, Niederman R. Evaluation of NSAIDs for treating post-endodontic pain. Endod Topics 2002;3:3–13.

Local anaesthesia

The most commonly used drugs in dentistry are the local anaesthetic drugs, which have been used since the late-1800s.

Local anaesthesia is a safe and effective method of pain control, and has a very low incidence of significant adverse effects. As a better understanding of the pharmacological dynamics of local anaesthetics has developed, the safety margin has improved. However, this increased safety should not change a clinician's perspective on the importance of understanding the pharmacology of the drug interactions and complications that can arise from local anaesthetic usage.

The most common mode of delivery for local anaesthesia in dentistry is via injection. The technique of injection depends on many factors. The two most commonly used injection techniques are infiltration and regional block:

- In **infiltration**, the effect of the anaesthetic is adjacent to the location of the injection.
- In **regional block**, the anaesthetic solution is injected adjacent to the nerve, but at a distance proximal to the site where anaesthesia is required. The aim is to prevent pain sensation for the entire nerve distribution distal to the site of injection.

Less commonly used injection techniques are intraligamentous and intraosseous injections. With **intraligamentous** injections, the solution is injected under pressure into the periodontal ligament. This approach is often used as a secondary approach to regional block or infiltration. An **intraosseous** injection utilises a small opening made through the cortical plate of the bone, and the local anaesthetic solution is injected directly into the underlying cancellous bone. It is used as a secondary approach to, for example, block or infiltration.

Local anaesthetic drugs currently in use do not cause vasoconstriction, therefore commonly a separate vasoconstrictor is added. The addition of a vasoconstrictor to a local anaesthetic solution allows a longer working time, and a reduced dose is required to achieve effective anaesthesia. A vasoconstrictor also reduces bleeding. Adrenaline and felypressin are the vasoconstrictors used most commonly (see p.49 and pp.52–3).

The maximum dose of local anaesthetic that can be used at one time depends on the local anaesthetic(s) used. See Table 6 (p.50) for maximum doses. If more than one local anaesthetic is used, the total dose used must be less than the maximum dose of the drug with the lower maximum dose. In dental practice, local anaesthetics are almost always given in single-use cartridges, with a usual volume of 2.2 mL.

It is essential to check that you are giving the correct drug (ie check the label on the cartridge) prior to injection.

Table 6 (p.50) summarises some of the characteristics of local anaesthetics. For adverse effects and toxic effects, see p.47.

Lignocaine hydrochloride without a vasoconstrictor is very short-acting and has limited applications in dentistry.

Drugs suitable for most dental procedures are:
- lignocaine hydrochloride with adrenaline
- prilocaine hydrochloride
- prilocaine hydrochloride with adrenaline
- articaine hydrochloride with adrenaline
- mepivacaine hydrochloride with adrenaline

Mepivacaine hydrochloride is useful for routine dental procedures of a short duration where the use of vasoconstrictors is contraindicated. Mepivacaine (with or without adrenaline) is suitable for use only in patients 3 years and older.

Articaine hydrochloride with adrenaline is suitable for use only in patients 4 years and older.

Bupivacaine hydrochloride with adrenaline is used for long surgical procedures where prolonged anaesthesia is required and for the management of postoperative pain. Its use should be restricted to patients 12 years and older.

POTENTIAL COMPLICATIONS OF LOCAL ANAESTHETICS

The most common complications with the use of local anaesthetic solutions are associated with anatomical or technique problems.

Difficulty in identifying anatomical landmarks (most commonly with inferior alveolar nerve blocks) can result in incomplete or failure of local anaesthetic effect. This is often associated with poor technique or anatomical variation.

Injecting local anaesthetic solution (particularly if it contains a vasoconstrictor) directly into the vascular system can cause significant systemic effects and increase the risk of adverse outcomes. See p.47 for systemic adverse effects of local anaesthetics.

Local complications

Relative to the number of local analgesic injections given nationally (and worldwide), the rates of complication (especially major complications) are exceedingly low.

There is a wide variety of potential local complications associated with local anaesthesia. These include equipment failure (eg needle breakage), anatomical issues (eg nerve trauma, paraesthesia, facial nerve paralysis), and tissue trauma—either operator- or patient-induced (eg trismus, haematoma, infection).

Nerve injuries resulting in paraesthesia or dysaesthesia are often considered a consequence of direct nerve trauma; however, some recent data suggest that there is a variation in chemoneurotoxicity of different local anaesthetic drugs. The literature is still limited in this area, and by far the more common effect is through direct nerve trauma, or through indirect nerve trauma from bleeding within the nerve sheath. The risk of nerve damage is greater if repeated injections are given into a previously partially anaesthetised site.

Trismus as a result of intramuscular injection of local anaesthetic drugs can occur, either as a direct effect of the drug, or as a result of bleeding within the muscle. When complications of prolonged anaesthesia or trismus occur, urgent specialist advice is indicated.

Although the local complications of local anaesthetic solution are generally not as significant as systemic complications, they can result in the patient needing to return for treatment, as well as loss of confidence in the operator. When complications are prolonged anaesthesia or trismus, urgent specialist advice is indicated.

FURTHER READING

Blanton PL, Jeske AH. Avoiding complications in local anesthesia induction: anatomical considerations. J Am Dent Assoc 2003; 134(7):888–93.

Malamed SF. Handbook of local anesthesia. 5th ed. St Louis: Mosby; 2004.

Medications in dentistry supplement. Aust Dent J 2005;50(4 Suppl 2): S1–81.

Roberts DH, Sowray JH. Local analgesia in dentistry. 3rd ed. Ch1–4; Bristol: Wright; 1987.

Oral sedation

Sedative and hypnotic drugs can be used for sedation of patients undergoing dental procedures to alleviate pain, fear and anxiety. This is often termed 'premedication'.

The oral route is the most commonly used route for drug administration; it is also the safest, most convenient and most economical. Oral sedation can be used quite effectively to reduce stress before and during dental treatment, and to manage preoperative and postoperative pain. It can be given the night before dental treatment to ensure restful sleep, or preoperatively to produce a light level of sedation that will lower preoperative anxiety.

The advantages and disadvantages of oral sedation are shown in Table 16.

ASSESSMENT OF PATIENTS FOR SEDATION

Patient selection and assessment is an essential prerequisite to the success of subsequent treatment under oral sedation. Careful pre-sedation appraisal optimises the safety and effectiveness of the sedation. The assessment is used to gain information from the patient to determine suitability for both sedation and dental treatment.

Table 16. Advantages and disadvantages of oral sedation

Advantages	Disadvantages
• almost universal acceptability • ease of administration • low cost • decreased incidence and severity of adverse effects compared with intravenous sedation • no need for needles, syringes, equipment • no need for specialised training	• reliance on patient adherence • long latent period • erratic and incomplete absorption • inability to titrate • inability to readily lighten or deepen the level of sedation • long duration of action

Pre-sedation appraisal must include asking for details of the nature of the patient's fears and anxieties, the medical, medication and dental histories, and information about social circumstances, including alcohol intake. Determine that the patient is fit for oral sedation.

Appropriate preoperative information and the patient's consent should be obtained. Patients should be aware of the effects of the drugs, including the possible adverse effects.

Alcohol should not be taken with any sedative.

PREPARATION OF PATIENTS FOR SEDATION

It is important that the patient is fully informed about the impact of all proposed treatment, the benefits of the treatment, its potential adverse effects, and the likely consequences of the action of a drug. The patient must consent to any procedures to be done under sedation before the sedation is given. (See Australian Dental Association website <http://www.ada.org.au> for further information about consent.)

Patients who are scheduled to receive oral sedation must be given careful verbal and written instruction as to their responsibility before and after sedation (see Box 15). The patient should arrange to be accompanied by a responsible adult who will act as escort and remain with the patient for the rest of the day. The patient should not eat or drink anything for two hours before their appointment time. The patient must not drive a vehicle, operate any machinery, drink alcohol, return to work, make any important decisions, or sign any important documents for 24 hours after the sedation.

DOSE OF DRUGS USED FOR SEDATION

After assessing the patient, the dose of drugs to be used for sedation can be determined; this requires particular attention to the medication history and alcohol intake. The response to sedatives is widely variable, and when prescribing a sedative, the patient's previous history must be considered.

Sedation used for **adults**:

1. *diazepam 5 to 10 mg orally, 1 hour before the procedure*

    OR

2. *temazepam 10 to 20 mg orally, 1 hour before the procedure.*

> **Box 15. Instructions for patients having oral sedation**
>
> **Before appointment**
>
> You must have nothing to eat or drink for 2 hours before your appointment time.
>
> If you are taking any medicines, they should be taken at the usual times.
>
> You will be given your oral sedative on arrival and will be asked to wait approximately 1 hour before your treatment commences.
>
> You should wear loose-fitting clothes, and no jewellery. Remove any contact lenses.
>
> You must be accompanied by a responsible adult who must remain in the waiting room throughout your appointment, escort you home afterwards and arrange for you to be looked after for the following 24 hours.
>
> Any illness occurring before the appointment should be reported immediately, as this might affect your treatment.
>
> **After sedation**
>
> You will remain at the clinic for at least 1 hour after your treatment has finished.
>
> Your escort must take you home (by other than public transport).
>
> You must rest and not undertake strenuous activities for the rest of the day.
>
> If you are hungry, you can have a light meal, but at lukewarm temperatures only.
>
> If you feel nauseated, you should sip a fizzy drink, then lie down.
>
> You must not drive any vehicle, operate any machinery or use any domestic appliance for 24 hours after the sedation.
>
> You must not drink alcohol, return to work, make any important decisions or sign any important documents for 24 hours after sedation.

MANAGEMENT

The semireclined (rather than fully reclined) position has less risk of airway contamination with blood, saliva, filling materials and teeth, and from passive reflux and aspiration. The patient should not be lying flat or head-down. The dental chair must be capable of being placed rapidly into the horizontal position for the purposes of cardiopulmonary resuscitation. Rubber dam should be used during all operative dental procedures to protect the airway. (See pp.172–5 for management of inhaled or swallowed objects.)

A pulse oximeter is a simple instrument that can be used to monitor the patient's pulse and arterial oxygen both during and following the procedure.

Patients should be observed by appropriately trained staff during the procedure and for at least one hour following the procedure before being discharged with their escort.

FURTHER READING

Guidelines on conscious sedation for dental procedures. Australian and New Zealand College of Anaesthetists and the Royal Australasian College of Dental Surgeons; 2003. <http://www.anzca.edu.au/pdfdocs/ps21_2003.pdf>.

Medical emergencies

The best way to avoid a medical emergency is by careful assessment of the patient; this includes obtaining a detailed medical and medication history.

Occasionally unavoidable emergencies occur. Prompt diagnosis and primary management can affect the outcome. Dental practitioners and their staff must be trained and have a plan for emergency management, so that a satisfactory outcome can be achieved.

> *A failed attempt at resuscitation is always better than failing to attempt resuscitation.*

Emergencies range from transient problems that resolve spontaneously (eg syncope), to medical emergencies that require the transfer of the patient to medical facilities (eg hypoglycaemia, severe asthma attack), to serious acute emergencies that require immediate on-site resuscitation (eg heart attack, anaphylactic reaction to drugs).

All drugs have the potential to cause adverse outcomes, some of which can be life-threatening (eg anaphylactic responses to penicillin occur approximately once every 10 000 courses administered, with 10% of these being fatal).

The information and guidelines in this chapter are *not* a substitute for formal training and regular updates. Valuable sources of information include the following:

- The *Therapeutic Guidelines* series has information on medical and medication-related problems.
- The Australian Resuscitation Council has policy statements and advice on resuscitation. Figure 7 (p. 187) is a basic life support flow chart that can be downloaded from the Australian Resuscitation Council website <http://www.resus.org.au/public/arc_basic_life_support.pdf>.

The *Therapeutic Guidelines* series and the Australian Resuscitation Council information form the basis of the following information.

CARDIOVASCULAR EMERGENCIES

Syncope

Syncope is a transient self-limiting loss of consciousness. The onset is almost always rapid, and the recovery is usually rapid, spontaneous and complete. The underlying mechanism for syncope is a transient global cerebral hypoperfusion. Presyncope refers to a condition in which the patient feels as though syncope is imminent, and symptoms tend to overlap premonitory symptoms of true syncope. In the presyncope phase, the patient feels light-headed, and may be nauseated and anxious; they may appear pale.

Syncopal episodes are common. The prevalence of syncope increases with age. Causes of syncope include neurally mediated syndromes (such as vasovagal/vasodepressor syncope), orthostatic syncope (including the effect of drugs and volume depletion), cardiac dysrhythmias (bradycardia and tachycardia), structural heart disease, and cerebrovascular disease.

The most common type of syncope in dental patients (and also generally) is vasovagal. This is usually a reaction to anxiety and fear before, during or after a dental procedure. Although a vasovagal attack is the most common cause of syncope, there *are* other causes and, particularly if recovery is slow or if the patient has had repeated events without obvious triggers, referral for medical evaluation is often necessary.

For management of syncope, see Box 16.

Coronary ischaemia

Coronary ischaemic syndromes are due to myocardial ischaemia secondary to coronary obstruction. A patient in the dental surgery may develop myocardial infarction, and it is imperative to identify this condition and have the patient transported to a hospital as swiftly as possible. Rapid identification of myocardial infarction and decisive action in referring the patient to appropriate care are essential to a good outcome.

Anginal pain is pain caused by temporary myocardial ischaemia resulting from a demand for more blood flow (most often due to exercise or emotional stress); it usually subsides promptly with rest as the increased demand subsides.

When a thrombus occludes a coronary artery so there is a vastly reduced blood flow beyond it, the result is severe myocardial ischaemia. The

> **Box 16. Management of syncope**
>
> If the patient feels faint:
> - Tilt the chair back to a horizontal position (the patient should not be placed in a 'head lower than heart' position).
> - Raise the patient's legs slightly.
> - Assess consciousness by talking to the patient.
>
> If the patient is unconscious:
> - Tilt the chair back to a horizontal position (the patient should not be placed in a 'head lower than heart' position).
> - Place the patient on their side (if they are pregnant, they should be turned to their left side).
> - Stimulate and cool the patient by placing a cold compress on their forehead.
>
> If the patient has a vasovagal-type syncope, they should rapidly return to consciousness; if they do not, they should be assessed for other causes of syncope or collapse.
>
> **Allow the patient to recover slowly under supervision; do not discharge them prematurely from care, particularly if they will be driving.**

ischaemia may produce an area of irritability within the myocardium which may produce life-threatening dysrhythmias (eg ventricular tachycardia, ventricular fibrillation). Both ventricular tachycardia and ventricular fibrillation may present as cardiac arrest. Death from cardiac arrest occurs rapidly.

If the coronary occlusion is not relieved, myocardial infarction develops progressively over the next 6 to 12 hours.

Angina

Angina typically presents as crushing chest pain in the centre of the chest, radiating to the left arm, and the neck or jaw. However, not all patients experience typical chest pain. Some experience atypical pain, or shortness of breath or light-headedness (angina equivalent).

A patient who is known to have episodes of angina should be instructed to bring their medication with them when they are presenting for dental treatment.

For management of angina, see Box 17 (p.168).

Box 17. Management of angina

Ensure any patient with a history of angina brings their medication (eg glyceryl trinitrate spray or tablets) when they attend for dental treatment.

If angina occurs:
- Cease dental treatment.
- Check pulse and level of consciousness.

The patient may be accustomed to treating their angina, and should have their medication with them.

- To shorten the attack, give:

    1 *glyceryl trinitrate spray 400-microgram metered dose sublingually, repeat the dose once after 5 minutes if pain persists (maximum of 2 metered doses)*

    OR

    1 *glyceryl trinitrate tablet 300 to 600 micrograms sublingually, repeat every 3 to 5 minutes if pain persists (to a maximum of 1800 micrograms)*

    OR

    1 *isosorbide dinitrate 5 mg sublingually, repeat every 5 minutes if pain persists (to a maximum of 15 mg).*

    Avoid nitrates if the patient has used sildenafil (Viagra) or vardenafil (Levitra) in the previous 24 hours, or tadalafil (Cialis) in the previous 5 days.

- Continue to monitor the patient, give reassurance, and give oxygen.

If the patient recovers, do not proceed with dental treatment; the patient should be medically evaluated even if apparently well.

If angina continues for more than 10 to 15 minutes, treat as for acute myocardial infarction.

Acute myocardial infarction

Myocardial infarction should be suspected if:
- chest pains similar to angina are unrelieved by up to 1800 micrograms glyceryl trinitrate tablets or 15 mg isosorbide dinitrate over 10 to 15 minutes, or 2 sprays of glyceryl trinitrate within 5 minutes

> **Box 18. Management of suspected acute myocardial infarction**
>
> Ensure any patient who has a history of angina brings their own medication (eg glyceryl trinitrate spray or tablets).
>
> - Call 000.
> - Monitor vital signs.
> - Give oxygen.
> - Give:
>
>   *aspirin 300 mg chewed or dissolved before swallowing.*
>
> - Unless the patient has just been taking glyceryl trinitrate spray or tablets or isosorbide dinitrate for angina, and provided they have not used sildenafil (Viagra) or vardenafil (Levitra) in the previous 24 hours, or tadalafil (Cialis) in the previous 5 days, give:
>
>   1 *glyceryl trinitrate spray 400-microgram metered dose sublingually, repeat the dose once after 5 minutes if pain persists (maximum of 2 metered doses)*
>
>   OR
>
>   1 *glyceryl trinitrate tablet 300 to 600 micrograms sublingually, repeat every 3 to 5 minutes if pain persists (to a maximum of 1800 micrograms)*
>
>   OR
>
>   1 *isosorbide dinitrate 5 mg sublingually, repeat every 5 minutes if pain persists (to a maximum of 15 mg).*
>
> - Continue to monitor and reassure until assistance arrives.
>
> **If the patient loses consciousness, institute basic life support—cardiopulmonary resuscitation (CPR)** (see Figure 7 'Basic life support flow chart', p.187). Use an automated external defibrillator if one is available.

- a patient with a history of angina says that the pain is much worse than usual
- this is the first ever episode of chest pain.

For management of a patient with suspected acute myocardial infarction, see Box 18.

Cardiac arrest

Cardiac arrest is generally due to ventricular tachycardia, ventricular fibrillation, asystole or electromechanical dissociation. The patient suddenly loses consciousness; there is no pulse, and no respiration.

See Box 19 for management of patients with cardiac arrest.

> **Box 19. Management of cardiac arrest**
> - Call 000.
> - Institute basic life support—cardiopulmonary resuscitation (CPR) (see Figure 7 'Basic life support flow chart', p.187).
> - Use an automated external defibrillator if one is available.
>
> Maintain treatment until patient regains consciousness or assistance arrives.

RESPIRATORY EMERGENCIES

Hyperventilation syndrome (gaseous alkalosis)

Hyperventilation syndrome may occur when a patient hyperventilates (overbreathes). It is common, and often occurs in patients suffering anxiety or an acute panic attack. Hyperventilation results in a lowering of the carbon dioxide level in the arterial blood which, if untreated, leads to a loss of drive of the respiratory centre.

Symptoms may include:
- light-headedness/dizziness
- shortness of breath
- a feeling of panic and impending death
- blurred vision
- tingling of the fingers, toes and lips
- a feeling of detachment.

Signs may include:
- rapid breathing
- occasional deep sighing breaths
- rapid pulse
- altered consciousness
- carpopedal spasm of the hands and fingers.

> **Box 20. Management of hyperventilation syndrome**
> - Encourage the patient to slow their breathing.
> - Have the patient rebreathe their expired air, by cupping their hands close over, but not obstructing, their mouth and nose.
> - Do *not* give oxygen (as this will prolong the symptoms).
>
> If there is not rapid recovery, the diagnosis should be reviewed and revised.
>
> If acute symptoms persist for more than 5 to 10 minutes, or if carpopedal spasm is extensive (and particularly if it spreads to involve the legs):
> - Call 000.

Symptoms of hyperventilation syndrome are commonly confused with syncope; they may also be the early phases of asthma or a heart attack.

Hyperventilation syndrome is best prevented by observing the patient (particularly following the administration of local anaesthetic, as hyperventilation syndrome commonly occurs at that time). If the patient is taking fast but shallow breaths, encourage them to slow their breathing and to breathe in through their nose and out through their mouth. Firmly reassure them, giving them an explanation of the cause of the symptoms, and have them talk to you.

See Box 20 for the management of patients with hyperventilation syndrome.

Acute asthma

Episodes of asthma can be fatal.

A patient who is known to have episodes of asthma should be instructed to bring their medication with them when they are presenting for dental treatment.

A rapid physical examination should be performed to evaluate the severity of the attack. See Table 17 (p.172) for assessment of severity of asthma in adults and children. Patients with severe asthma may have no wheeze. Patients with cyanosis require prompt hospitalisation.

Wheezing is an unreliable indicator of the severity of an asthma attack and may be absent in a severe attack.

Cyanosis indicates life-threatening asthma.

For management of acute asthma, see Box 21 (p.173).

Table 17. Initial assessment of the severity of an acute attack of asthma

Clinical features	Mild	Moderate	Severe and life-threatening
physical exhaustion / altered conscious state	no	no	yes
increased accessory muscle use (in children)	no	some	marked
talks in	sentences	phrases	words
pulse rate*	<100/minute	*adults*: 100–120/minute *children*: 100–200/minute	*adults*: >120/minute *children*: >200/minute
hospital admission needed	no	probably, especially if poor initial treatment response	yes, consider ICU

* bradycardia (slow pulse rate) may be seen when respiratory arrest is imminent

Inhaled or swallowed objects

There is always a risk of objects being inhaled or swallowed during dental treatment. An inhaled or swallowed object may present a significant risk to the patient's health and wellbeing. Foreign objects in the lungs (inhaled objects) must be removed as a matter of urgency. Swallowed objects may have an uneventful passage through the gastrointestinal tract; occasionally they may need to be removed. There may be medicolegal implications for the practitioner in the event of an object becoming lodged in the lungs or the gastrointestinal tract.

Prevention of inhaled or swallowed objects

All steps must be taken to minimise the risk of accidental inhalation or swallowing of foreign objects:

- When practicable, a rubber dam should be used for procedures where the risk of inhalation or swallowing is high.
- If procedures preclude the use of rubber dam, precautions to take include
  - ensuring a careful and unrushed approach
  - having the patient reclined rather than supine

> **Box 21. Management of acute asthma**
>
> Ensure that any patient who has a history of asthma brings the bronchodilator medication they use to treat attacks.
>
> The initial management of an asthma attack is determined by the severity of this attack (see Table 17), and the patient's background asthma pattern and severity.
>
> If the attack of asthma is **mild**:
> - Cease dental treatment.
> - Give 4 puffs of a bronchodilator (eg salbutamol) (preferably via a spacer).
> - Wait 4 minutes.
> - Give a further 4 puffs of the bronchodilator, if necessary.
> - Wait 4 minutes.
>
> Assess status of the patient. If the patient recovers swiftly:
> - Temporise the dental state.
> - Make another appointment to complete the treatment (if needed).
> - When the patient is breathing easily, discharge from care.
> - Recommend that the patient takes medications strictly as prescribed and, if that is not effective, has a medical review.
>
> If the attack of asthma is **moderate or severe**:
> - Call 000.
> - Cease dental treatment.
> - Give 4 puffs of a bronchodilator (eg salbutamol) (preferably via a spacer).
> - Wait 4 minutes.
> - Give a further 4 puffs of the bronchodilator.
> - Wait 4 minutes.
> - Give oxygen continuously.
> - Make another appointment to complete the treatment.
>
> Continue to monitor the patient until assistance arrives.

- having instruments and facilities available that can be used to retrieve an object from the oropharynx
- (if appropriate) tying floss to any object that can be dropped
- placing gauze across the back of the tongue to trap small items (eg crowns) that may be dropped
- rotating the patient's head so that a dropped object will fall to the side of the mouth
- using high-volume suction.

Table 18. Signs of obstruction

Partial obstruction	Complete obstruction
wheeze	inability to breath, speak, cry or cough
stridor (noisy inspiration)	agitation, gripping of the throat
laboured breathing	cyanosis
coughing spasms	bulging of the neck veins
cyanosis (indicates a severe lack of oxygen)	rapid development of respiratory failure (followed by cardiac failure)
	loss of consciousness

Obstruction of the airway

It is important to differentiate between partial and complete airway obstruction following accidental inhalation of a foreign body. If the patient can breathe, speak, cry or cough, some movement of air is occurring, and the obstruction is partial. See Table 18 for signs of partial and complete obstruction.

For management of a patient with an inhaled or swallowed object, see Box 22.

Box 22. Management of an inhaled or swallowed object*

In the event that an object appears to disappear down the oropharynx:
- Cease the dental procedure.
- Check the patient's vital signs.
- Check whether the object is present in the patient's mouth or clothes and, if so, remove it.
- If the object is not found, put the patient into an upright position.
- Do not allow the patient to drink.
- Arrange for a chest radiograph (as a swallowed object will remain in the upper gastrointestinal tract for some time, a chest radiograph done within one hour will show any radiopaque object that has been inhaled or swallowed; if the time interval is longer, a swallowed object will have passed through the upper gastrointestinal tract).
- If the patient is coughing, encourage them to relax, breathe deeply and try to dislodge the object by the coughing. Look at all spit and expectorant for the foreign body.

continued next page

Box 22. Management of an inhaled or swallowed object* (cont.)

All objects in the lungs should be removed by bronchoscopy or thoracotomy, and sharp objects such as needles or endodontic files in the gastrointestinal tract should be removed by gastroscopy, colonoscopy or laparotomy.

If **partial obstruction** (see Table 18) is present:
- Call 000

Remain with the patient to reassure them and to encourage them to cough up the foreign body.

If **total obstruction** (see Table 18) is present:
- Call 000.
- Turn patient on to their side.
- Attempt to clear and open the airway by manually removing the obstruction.

Check for signs of breathing. If no signs of breathing:
- Give 5 back blows between the shoulder blades using the heel of the hand (checking for effectiveness between each blow).

Check for signs of breathing. If no signs of breathing:
- Give 5 chest thrusts (checking for effectiveness between each thrust) (chest thrusts are identical to cardiac compressions but sharper and harder).

If total obstruction continues:
- Cricothyroidotomy is indicated
  - Extend the head back to stretch the neck.
  - Palpate the cricothyroid ligament.
  - Incise through the skin and ligament, or place a large-bore needle.
  - Maintain airway until help arrives.

(Note: The Heimlich manoeuvre, which is a technique to apply abdominal thrust to expel an airway foreign body, is currently not recommended by the Australian Resuscitation Council. This is on the basis that it can damage internal organs [particularly the liver, spleen and stomach], it may precipitate regurgitation of stomach contents, and it is dangerous for pregnant women.)

---

* A flow chart for the management of choking can be downloaded from the Australian Resuscitation Council website <http://www.resus.org.au/public/arc_choking.pdf>.

NEUROLOGICAL EMERGENCIES

Stroke

The signs and symptoms of transient ischemic attack or stroke may include:
- transient loss of consciousness
- difficulty of movement of one side of the body
- confusion
- difficulty in speaking.

For management of patient with an acute stroke, see Box 23.

Box 23. Management of stroke

- Call 000.
- Administer oxygen.
- Maintain airway.

Monitor the patient's vital signs until assistance arrives. It is difficult to identify whether the stroke is haemorrhagic or ischaemic; therefore, aspirin should *not* be given.

Seizures

Patients with epilepsy can have seizures during dental treatment or while in the dental practitioner's office. Not all fitting is epileptic; patients suffering syncope, hypoglycaemia, stroke and cerebral hypoxia from other causes can present with seizures. Children with fever can have seizures.

Seizures can take many forms. They can be generalised or partial. There can be:
- warning symptoms (aura)
- a sudden spasm of muscles (producing rigidity such that the patient falls)
- jerky movements of the head, arms and legs
- loss of consciousness (which may be associated with noisy breathing, salivation and urinary incontinence).

In status epilepticus, recurrent seizures occur without recovery of consciousness between attacks. This is a medical emergency and the patient should be swiftly transferred to hospital.

See Box 24 for management of patients with seizures.

> **Box 24. Management of seizures**
>
> The first priority in the management of a patient having a seizure is to ensure that the patient is not in danger in the dental chair:
> - Protect the patient from falling from the chair and injuring themselves on surrounding equipment, or lift them onto the floor.
> - Avoid restraining the patient during the seizure unless it is essential to avoid injury.
> - Wait until obvious fitting has subsided.
> - Check conscious state.
> - Maintain airway.
> - Check for breathing.
> - If there is vomitus, remove it from the mouth and pharynx by high-volume suction.
>
> If the seizure or loss of consciousness lasts for more than a few minutes:
> - Call 000.
>
> Remain with the patient until help arrives.
>
> If the patient recovers completely, they should be kept under observation for at least a further 30 minutes. They must not be allowed to drive home by themselves, and should be advised to seek urgent medical review.
>
> If recurrent seizures occur without recovery of consciousness between attacks:
> - Protect the airway.
> - Call 000.

ENDOCRINE EMERGENCIES

Endocrine problems can cause a wide range of medical emergencies. Generally, in the dental setting, an endocrine emergency occurs only in a patient with a known history of an endocrine disorder.

Diabetes

Hypoglycaemia

Hypoglycaemia in patients on insulin or insulin secretogogues occurs when the blood glucose level falls low enough to cause symptoms and signs (ie less than 3 to 5 mmol/L). There are two groups of symptoms of hypoglycaemia:
- those mediated by the sympathetic nervous system (adrenergic symptoms)

- pale skin
- sweating
- shaking
- palpitations
- feeling of anxiety
- those due to altered brain function (neuroglycopenic symptoms)
    - hunger
    - suboptimal intellectual function
    - confusion and inappropriate behaviour
    - coma
    - seizures.

Hypoglycaemia can occur at any time of the day or night. Factors that increase the risk of hypoglycaemia include inappropriately high doses of insulin or insulin secretogogue, forgotten or delayed meals, insufficient carbohydrate (especially if taking rapid-acting insulins or insulin secretogogues), and unaccustomed or unplanned exercise.

See Box 25 for management of patients with hypoglycaemia.

> **Box 25. Management of hypoglycaemia**
>
> If the patient is **conscious and cooperative**:
> - Defer dental treatment.
> - Give a sugar-containing food (eg fruit juice, jelly beans, honey). This must be followed by a longer-acting carbohydrate (eg sandwich, dried fruit).
>
> Normal diabetic therapy should not be interrupted.
>
> A patient who has mild hypoglycaemia should remain under supervision until they feel recovered. They should not drive themselves home, and they should be strongly advised to seek medical advice.
>
> If the patient is **drowsy or uncooperative, or unconscious**:
> - Call 000.

Diabetic ketoacidosis

Diabetic ketoacidosis occurs primarily in patients with type 1 diabetes and is characterised by:
- hyperglycaemia
- polyuria
- polydipsia
- hyperventilation

- dehydration.

Infection, trauma and, in adolescents, omission of insulin are common precipitants of ketoacidosis in patients with type 1 diabetes.

Diabetic ketoacidosis is a medical emergency requiring specialist medical care (see Box 26).

> **Box 26. Management of diabetic ketoacidosis**
> - Call 000.
> - Organise transport to medical facilities.

Addisonian (adrenal) crisis

Addisonian (adrenal) crisis can present 6 to 12 hours after surgical stress in a patient taking corticosteroids who has not had them increased before the surgery. (See pp.74–5 for management of patients on corticosteroids.)

As there is a lag time before the onset of an Addisonian crisis, there is a risk that it may occur silently when the patient is at home in bed. Consequently, it is recommended that patients taking corticosteroids are treated in the morning, so that if symptoms occur, they will present when they are normally awake.

An Addisonian crisis is a medical emergency and patients should be treated in an emergency department or hospital (see Box 27 for management).

> **Box 27. Management of Addisonian (adrenal) crisis**
> - Call 000.
>
> The patient will require corticosteroids.
> - If the patient is **rousable and can swallow**, give them their own corticosteroid tablets (hydrocortisone or prednis(ol)one).
> - If the patient is **unconscious and help is not immediately available**, give
>
>   *hydrocortisone 200 mg IM or IV.*

ALLERGIES

A patient who is known to have an allergy should be instructed to bring their medication with them when they are presenting for dental treatment.

Causes

Antibiotic hypersensitivity

A history of allergy, particularly to penicillin, must be specifically checked for before prescribing a beta-lactam antibiotic (eg phenoxymethylpenicillin, cephalexin). A patient with a known beta-lactam hypersensitivity should be encouraged to wear an alert bracelet or necklace containing this information.

See p.15 for a discussion about antibiotic hypersensitivity, and pp.181–7 for management.

Latex allergy

Latex allergy is rare. If a patient claims to be allergic to latex, they should be referred to a specialist to confirm their condition. Dental treatment should be performed only in a specialist centre. Latex allergy usually presents as a localised urticarial or eczematous contact reaction starting minutes to hours after exposure. Occasionally it may present as a life-threatening systemic reaction. A dental practitioner, staff member or patient who shows evidence of a possible latex allergy should be investigated by a clinical immunologist. An affected person should be encouraged to wear an alert bracelet or necklace and, if there is a significant risk of exposure, carry adrenaline in case of a severe anaphylactic reaction.

If contact dermatitis occurs on the patient's face following dental surgery, the possibility of latex allergy must be considered. It can be avoided by the dental practitioner using 'latex-free' gloves and rubber dam. If there is a severe reaction, the patient should be treated as for anaphylaxis (see Box 29, p.138, and Box 30, pp.184–7).

Allergic reaction to local anaesthetics

Allergic reactions to local anaesthetics are rare—the most common causes of abnormal symptoms following local anaesthetic injections are syncope and hyperventilation.

An intravascular injection of adrenaline can cause breathlessness, throbbing headache, pallor, rapid pulse and palpitations. Patients generally respond rapidly to supportive care.

Patients may experience an allergic reaction to components in the local anaesthetic solution; however, this now occurs infrequently because stabilisers have been removed from the anaesthetic solution. There is a theoretical risk of an allergic reaction to the latex of the bung in a cartridge, but this has not been reported clinically.

If a patient indicates that they are allergic to local anaesthetic, their previous history must be discussed carefully with them. There are rare cases of true allergy to local anaesthetic; patients show either an urticarial or eczematous response, or a true anaphylactic reaction. If an allergy to local anaesthetic is suspected, the patient should be referred to a specialist immunologist or anaesthetist with training in drug reactions to check the nature of the response.

True allergic reactions should be treated as for allergy (see Box 28, p.182) or anaphylactic reaction (see pp.182–7).

Food allergy

Although food allergy is relatively rare, there is a significant number of individuals suffering from allergies to food (including fish, nuts, eggs and dairy [in children]), and food substances (eg preservatives). Such individuals may present at dental surgeries after being exposed *en route*.

Types of allergic reactions

Several different reaction mechanisms produce urticarial drug eruptions and angioedema that show similar clinical features.

Urticaria

Urticaria is characterised by transient erythematous raised oedematous wheals that move and may coalesce to take on unusual shapes. Scratching or pressure can worsen or trigger the lesions. Many drug-associated eruptions begin towards the end of an antibiotic course (day 4 to 10 after starting therapy); some may start earlier (see 'Anaphylactic and anaphylactoid reactions', p.182).

Where a drug is suspected or established as the cause of urticaria, removal may be the solution. However, even when this is done, the urticaria may not immediately cease. Occasionally, external contact with certain substances causes urticaria (contact urticaria) and removing contact with the cause (eg latex rubber gloves) may control the problem.

Treatment of acute urticaria depends on the severity. See Box 28 (p.182) for management of patients with urticaria.

> **Box 28. Management of urticaria**
>
> For **mild urticaria**:
> - Give an oral antihistamine. Use a less sedating agent during the day (eg cetirizine, fexofenadine, loratadine) and, if required, a sedating agent at night (eg pheniramine, promethazine).
>
> Patients with **extensive urticaria**, or **severe urticaria involving eyelids and lips** need referral for urgent medical attention.
>
> If there is associated hypotension and evidence of anaphylactic shock:
> - Call 000.
> - Give adrenaline (see Box 29, p.183, and Box 30, pp.184–7, for management of anaphylactic reaction).

Angioedema

Acute oedema of the subcutaneous tissue, either as single or multiple lesions, is typical of angioedema. Lesions are not itchy and may occur anywhere, but frequently affect the face, periorbital region, lips, tongue, glottis, dorsa of feet and hands, and genitalia. Individual lesions resolve over hours to several days.

Angioedema can be painful or burning, and is particularly dramatic when it causes swelling of the lips, eyelids or tongue. Laryngeal involvement can cause airway obstruction. Drug causation should be considered, particularly in cases of acute urticaria and angioedema.

Angioedematous lesions are common in acute and chronic forms of urticaria. Treatment is the same as for urticaria (see Box 28).

Anaphylactic and anaphylactoid reactions

Anaphylactic (IgE-mediated) and anaphylactoid (pseudoallergic) reactions have overlapping clinical features. Anaphylactic and anaphylactoid reactions usually appear within minutes of parenteral or mucosal exposure to a drug, and around 30 minutes to hours after drug ingestion.

> **Box 29. Management of anaphylactoid and anaphylactic reactions***
>
> A patient who is known to have an allergy should be instructed to bring their medication with them when they are presenting for dental treatment.
>
> If an anaphylactoid or anaphylactic reaction occurs:
> - Call 000.
> - Remove and/or cease allergen.
> - Cease dental treatment.
> - Give adrenaline (in doses shown in Box 30, pp.184–5, for management of anaphylactic reaction), either
>   - autoinjector into the anterolateral thigh (through clothes if necessary), or tongue
>
>   OR
>   - drawn-up solution into the anterolateral thigh, tongue or floor of mouth.
> - Give oxygen.
>
> If patient loses consciousness:
> - Institute basic life support—cardiopulmonary resuscitation (CPR) (see 'Basic life support flow chart', p.187).
>
> Maintain treatment until assistance arrives.
>
> * The full medical management of severe anaphylactoid and anaphylactic reactions is given in Box 30 (pp.184–7).

Anaphylactic urticaria and angioedema begin soon after drug exposure. Other features of anaphylaxis include bronchospasm, laryngeal oedema, abdominal cramps, diarrhoea and hypotension.

Anaphylactoid urticaria and angioedema with or without hypotension and bronchospasm similarly present soon after drug administration. Itch and/or urticaria alone can occur in milder presentations, and are more often seen after oral administration; they are occasionally seen following subcutaneous or intramuscular administration.

See Box 29 (above) and Box 30 (pp.184–7) for management of patients with anaphylactoid or anaphylactic reactions.

Box 30. Medical management of severe anaphylactoid and anaphylactic reactions*

Clinical recognition

Early
- sensations of warmth, itching especially in axillae and groins
- feelings of anxiety or panic

Progressive
- erythematous or urticarial rash
- oedema of face, neck, soft tissues

Severe
- hypotension (shock)
- bronchospasm (wheezing)
- laryngeal oedema (dyspnoea, stridor, aphonia, drooling)
- arrhythmias, cardiac arrest

   Note: The onset of severe clinical features may be extremely rapid without prodromal features.

Acute management

A severe anaphylactoid reaction is a life-threatening emergency.

As in all medical emergencies, initial management should be directed at the ABC of resuscitation, namely: Airway, Breathing and Circulation. If working alone, call for assistance.

1. Cease administration of any suspected medication or diagnostic contrast material immediately, remove allergen from patient's mouth, scrape out bee stings.
2. Administer oxygen by face mask at 6–8 L/minute.
3. **Adults**

   Inject adrenaline **1:1000 intramuscularly**:

   small adults (less than 50 kg) give 0.25 mL

   average adults (50–100 kg) give 0.50 mL

   large adults (more than 100 kg) give 0.75 mL

continued next page

Box 30. Medical management of severe anaphylactoid and anaphylactic reactions* (cont.)

Children (up to 25 kg)

Use adrenaline **1:10 000**
or
dilute 1 ampoule (1 mL) of adrenaline 1:1000 with 9 mL water for injection or normal saline.

Inject **intramuscularly** up to a maximum of 500 micrograms (5 mL) according to the guide (**approximates to 10 micrograms/kg**).

1 year (10 kg) give 1 mL

3 years (15 kg) give 1.5 mL

5 years (20 kg) give 2 mL

8 years (25 kg) give 2.5 mL

Children more than 25 kg, as for small adults

Note: Approximate body weight may be calculated by the formula $(2 \times Age) + 9 = $ weight in kg.

4. Establish one, or preferably two, wide-bore intravenous lines (16 gauge or larger). Commence rapid fluid resuscitation with normal saline or Hartmann's solution.
5. If there is severe laryngospasm, bronchospasm, circulatory shock or coma, intubate and commence intermittent positive pressure ventilation.
6. If there has been little or no response to the initial intramuscular dose of adrenaline, administer 5 micrograms/kg slowly into the intravenous line. Repeat at 5-minute intervals depending on response. If the patient remains shocked, start an adrenaline infusion (preferably via a central venous line), commencing at 0.25 micrograms/kg/minute, and titrating as required to restore blood pressure. Large doses of adrenaline may be needed.

Additional measures

- Beta$_2$ agonists for bronchospasm: administer salbutamol or terbutaline by aerosol or nebuliser.
- Antihistamines: administer both H$_1$- and H$_2$-receptor blockers slowly intravenously:
  promethazine 0.5 to 1 mg/kg
  AND
  ranitidine 1 mg/kg or famotidine 0.4 mg/kg or cimetidine 4 mg/kg.

continued next page

Box 30. Medical management of severe anaphylactoid and anaphylactic reactions* (cont.)

- Corticosteroids: administer intravenously:
  hydrocortisone 2 to 6 mg/kg or dexamethasone 0.1–0.4 mg/kg.
- Nebulised adrenaline (5 mL of 1:1000) may be tried in laryngeal oedema and often will ease upper airways obstruction. However, do not delay intubation if upper airways obstruction is progressive.

Supportive treatment

- Observe vital signs frequently and, if possible, monitor electrocardiogram and pulse oximetry.
- All patients who have suffered a severe anaphylactoid reaction must be admitted to hospital. Patients who remain clinically unstable after initial resuscitation should be admitted to an intensive care unit.
- If patients are not admitted to hospital, for example if they respond to first treatment, provide information to them in case of a possible late reaction.

Notes

1. The mainstay in the treatment of severe anaphylaxis is the prompt use of adrenaline which can be lifesaving. Withholding adrenaline due to misplaced concerns of possible adverse effects can result in deterioration and death of the patient. Adrenaline must be used at the first suspicion of anaphylaxis. It is safe and effective.
2. All ampoules of adrenaline contain 1 mg (1000 micrograms). Adrenaline 1:1000 contains 1 mg in 1 mL (ie 1000 micrograms/mL), whereas adrenaline 1:10 000 contains 1 mg in 10 mL (ie 100 micrograms/mL).
   Either concentration may be used intramuscularly or injected into a fast flowing intravenous infusion. If injected directly into a vein, only the 1:10 000 strength should be used (or 1 mL of 1:1000 diluted with 9 mL normal saline).
   The initial dose of adrenaline is 5 micrograms/kg (children 10 micrograms/kg). The repeat dose for adults and children is 5 micrograms/kg. The volume doses given in 'Acute management' are an approximation to this and are appropriate in acute emergency situations to avoid unnecessary delays.
3. Although additional vasopressor agents are rarely needed, occasional cases are resistant to adrenaline—especially if the patient is taking beta blocking drugs. If adrenaline in adequate doses is not improving the situation, give glucagon 1 mg intravenously and consider changing to a noradrenaline infusion.
4. If anaesthesia is required for intubation, use fentanyl 1 to 10 micrograms/kg intravenously. Care should be taken if using thiopentone, midazolam or propofol as these drugs will exacerbate hypotension. Suxamethonium 1 to 2 mg/kg may be used to facilitate intubation, but should be used *only* if the operator is sure of being able to intubate. Cricoid pressure should be applied during laryngoscopy and intubation.
5. Corticosteroids and antihistamines may modify the overall duration of a reaction and may prevent relapse. However, onset of action will be delayed and they must never be used to the exclusion of adrenaline.

continued next page

> **Box 30. Medical management of severe anaphylactoid and anaphylactic reactions* (cont.)**
>
> 6. Some drugs and intravenous fluids used in the treatment of anaphylactoid reactions may themselves cause such a reaction. This includes intravenous antihistamines and corticosteroids. Reactions to these substances are rare and should not preclude their use unless the patient has had a known previous reaction to them.
> 7. Less severe reactions can only be classified in retrospect. Therefore administration of adrenaline should not be delayed.
> 8. All patients should be followed up for investigation of possible provoking factors and further management.
>
> * This chart has been reproduced with permission from Australian Prescriber. It was published as an insert to Australian Prescriber 2001, Vol. 24, No. 5. The chart has been updated and endorsed by the Australasian College for Emergency Medicine, the Australian Society of Clinical Immunology and Allergy, the Australian and New Zealand College of Anaesthetists, the Royal Australasian College of Physicians, the Royal Australian and New Zealand College of Radiologists, and the Royal Australian College of General Practitioners.

Figure 7. Basic life support flow chart*

D — Check for **Danger**

hazards / risks / safety?

R — **Responsive?** (unconscious?)

If not, call for help
Call 000 / resuscitation team

A — Open **Airway**
Look for signs of life (conscious, responsive, breathing normally, moving)

B — Give 2 initial **Breaths** if not breathing normally

C — Give 30 chest **Compressions** (almost 2 compressions/second) followed by 2 breaths

D — Attach automated external **Defibrillator** as soon as available and follow its prompts

Continue **CPR** (cardiopulmonary resuscitation) until qualified personnel arrive or signs of life return

* Adapted from the Australian Resuscitation Council flow chart. The flow chart can be downloaded from the Australian Resuscitation Council website <http://www.resus.org.au/public/arc_basic_life_support.pdf>.

EMERGENCY DRUGS AND EQUIPMENT

There is conflicting advice from various organisations and texts as to the extent of emergency equipment that a dental practitioner should have available to assist in the management of medical emergencies in dental patients. These range from virtually no equipment to a full emergency doctor's bag. One of the difficulties is that, usually and hopefully, medical emergencies in dental surgeries are uncommon, and there is risk that medications will have expired before being needed; this is either easily overlooked or expensive.

All dental practitioners have a professional obligation to ensure that they are properly trained and are up to date with emergency management. This includes ensuring that all staff are correctly trained in emergency management, and have maintained their competence. If dental assistants have not been through a formal training program, they should have, at least, a basic level first aid certificate.

There should be an established plan for obtaining medical assistance. The emergency number (000) for calling paramedical services should be prominently placed, and also the number of the nearest available medical facility. The reasonable time that medical assistance can arrive needs to be known; thus, for example, a dental clinic as part of the wider health clinic involving medical and nursing practitioners could reasonably expect assistance within a matter of minutes, whereas for an isolated suburban or rural practice, a reasonable response time may be more than 30 minutes.

Generally, the longer the time before assistance can reasonably be expected to arrive, the greater the need for staff training and equipment.

Drugs and equipment required by dental practitioners for emergencies

Dental practitioners should carefully consider their emergency equipment needs and staff training, relevant to their location, patient population and practice type.

The **minimum requirements** for emergency situations in the dental surgery are oxygen, a disposable airway, and adrenaline.

- **Oxygen**: All surgeries should have an oxygen source which can be easily transported to the patient. The simplest and safest way of administering oxygen to a patient who is not breathing is via a bag/mask/valve supplemented with oxygen at 6 to 8 L/minute. Oxygen-powered resuscitators are not recommended as there is risk of gaseous extension of the stomach resulting in regurgitation. Relative analgesia machines with the oxygen override are not an efficient means of administering oxygen, and do not allow ventilation of the patient who is not breathing.

- **Airway**: Simple disposable plastic airways secure the oral airway, and facilitate mouth-to-mouth resuscitation or ventilation with oxygen.
- **Adrenaline**: Adrenaline should be available to be injected into the tongue or anterolateral thigh. Adrenaline is available in ampoules (1:1000 and 1:10 000), and pre-loaded syringes (1:1000 and 1:2000). A pre-loaded syringe is preferred to a vial, since the latter requires preparation and needs to be drawn up into a syringe—this can be difficult and time-consuming with a severe anaphylactic emergency when few staff may be available. There must be sufficient quantities of adrenaline in the surgery to be able to give two doses.

There is a second level of **medications that are considered desirable**:

- **Glucose**: Patients exhibiting signs of hypoglycaemia require a readily available glucose-containing food (eg fruit juice, jelly beans, honey).
- **Glyceryl trinitrate tablet or spray**: Patients with a history of angina usually have their tablets with them and administer their usual dose sublingually. However, it is suggested that the dental emergency kit include glyceryl trinitrate spray (which has a much longer shelf-life than tablets), in case the patient does not have their glyceryl trinitrate.
- **Bronchodilator** (eg salbutamol) and **spacer**: Patients with a history of asthma usually have their inhaler with them, and can administer their usual treatment if necessary. It is suggested that the dental practitioner could have a bronchodilator available for a patient who has not brought their own inhaler.
- **Aspirin**: Aspirin may be required for a patient with suspected acute myocardial infarction.
- **Hydrocortisone** for injection: Hydrocortisone may be required for patients with an Addisonian crisis. It may also be used in the management of anaphylactic and anaphylactoid reactions.

There are other medical equipment **items that may be useful** in the dental surgery, depending on the nature of the practice:

- A **blood pressure monitor** is useful for assessment of cardiovascular patients and collapsed patients.

- A **blood glucose monitor** is useful in the assessment of patients with diabetes.
- A **pulse oximeter** is essential if intravenous sedation procedures are performed, and is desirable for oral sedative procedures.
- **Laryngeal airways** provide a substantial level of airway protection and minimise the risk of gastric insufflation. They also make ventilating the patient easier, allowing any member of staff to assist in intermittent positive pressure ventilation.
- The simplicity and effectiveness of **automated external defibrillators** has resulted in their widespread availability in ambulances, hospital outpatient departments, airports and major shopping malls.

FURTHER READING

Guidelines at Australian Resuscitation Council Online <http://www.resus.org.au/>.

Malamed S. Medical emergencies in the dental office. 5th ed. St Louis: Mosby; 2000.

Appendix 1
Drugs and sport

Sporting authorities have requirements regarding drugs that are prohibited for competitors in sporting events. Some of the drugs prohibited in sport may be prescribed or administered by dentists for dental treatment.

If drugs are required to treat an elite athlete, care must be taken regarding which drugs are used or prescribed. Most elite athletes are very aware of the requirements for their particular sport.

Each national sporting federation or association has an antidoping policy that will have a list of prohibited substances. Most sporting bodies reference the World Anti-Doping Code's prohibited list <http://www.wada-ama.org/en/prohibitedlist.ch2>, which is maintained by the World Anti-Doping Agency (WADA). The prohibited list includes categories and specific substances that are prohibited in sport. A substance that is not specifically listed may nonetheless be banned, as it may belong to a category on the list, or it may contain a derivative of a prohibited substance. The list is reviewed and updated annually. The list is divided into substances and methods that are prohibited at all times, and those that are prohibited during competitions only.

Drug groups on the prohibited list include:
- anabolic steroids (eg testosterone)
- hormones and related substances (eg growth hormone)
- antioestrogen drugs (eg tamoxifen)
- diuretics and other masking agents (eg frusemide, thiazides, probenecid)
- stimulants (eg amphetamine)
- narcotics (eg morphine, oxycodone)
- cannabinoids (eg marijuana)
- glucocorticoids (eg prednisolone).

Information about drugs and their status for sporting participants can be ascertained from the Australian Sports Anti-Doping Authority (ASADA), 1800 020 506 <http://www.asada.gov.au/substances/>, and from WADA <http://www.wada-ama.org/en/>.

Appendix 2
Dental procedures and drugs during pregnancy and breastfeeding

Most dental treatment can be carried out with safety during pregnancy.

Elective procedures requiring general anaesthesia or intravenous sedation should be deferred until after the baby is born and, preferably, until breastfeeding has been ceased. If the patient is unsure whether she is pregnant, the decision about whether to proceed should be deferred until this is known. In general, elective treatment is best performed in the second trimester (ie the fourth, fifth and sixth months) of pregnancy.

If dental radiographs are necessary for assessment or diagnosis of infection or trauma, or for treatment of these conditions, there is no reason, on radiation protection grounds, to defer them. The Australian Radiation Protection and Nuclear Safety Agency (ARPANSA) guidelines* state that there are no contraindications to the taking of intraoral radiographs during pregnancy; however, provision of a leaded drape is recommended when the X-ray beam is directed downwards towards the patient's trunk (eg when taking occlusal views of the maxilla).

Pregnancy and the use of drugs

A drug can have more than one harmful effect on the fetus. Individual effects depend on the time of fetal exposure to the drug.

During the first two weeks after fertilisation and prior to full implantation, the embryo is thought to be resistant to any teratogenic effects of drugs. This is because there is no direct communication between maternal and embryonic tissue until after the placenta starts to form.

The critical period with respect to teratogenic effects is during organogenesis. This starts at about 17 days after conception and is complete by 60 to 70 days. Exposure to certain drugs during this period (17 to 70 days) can cause major birth defects.

---

* *Radiation protection in dentistry: Radiation protection series No. 10. Australian Radiation Protection and Nuclear Safety Agency; December 2005.*

Some drugs can interfere with functional development of organ systems (eg central nervous system, integumentary system, cardiovascular system) in the second and third trimesters and produce serious consequences.

It is quite possible that a woman may not be aware of her pregnancy until after the early stages of organogenesis. For this reason, drugs in the most severe category of risk (Category X in the Australian categorisation below) should not be prescribed to a woman of childbearing potential, unless a pregnancy test is negative and she is using an effective method of contraception.

However, there are several conditions in which long-term medication may be necessary in a woman of childbearing potential despite known risks of the drugs. At the time of initial prescribing in any such situation, the prescriber should discuss the desirability of reviewing medication requirements well before conception. For some disorders, it may be possible to change to a different category of drug. If a patient conceives while on medication and there has been no opportunity for prior discussion with the prescriber, her medication should be reviewed as soon as possible.

The following check list may assist in deciding whether to prescribe a particular drug during pregnancy:

- **Nonpharmacological interventions**: Is such an intervention available and likely to be successful? Would such an intervention be reasonable at least until the first trimester is complete? Most pregnant women strongly favour this type of intervention and compliance is likely to be high.
- **Risk–benefit analysis**: For the particular drug under consideration, what are the potential risks and benefits of prescribing to the mother, and risks to the fetus? What are the risks and benefits (to each) of *not* prescribing?
- **Incidence of spontaneous congenital abnormality**: Where medication cannot be avoided, it may be appropriate to discuss the incidence of non–drug-related, spontaneous abnormalities. This is often underestimated. The incidence in Australia of significant congenital abnormality is 2% to 4% of live births, and minor abnormalities are recognised in approximately 15% of newborns.
- **Education, documentation and communication**: Has the education of the woman and her partner regarding risks and benefits been properly documented in the patient's notes? Have those health professionals involved in obstetric management been informed?

Routine review later in the pregnancy includes consideration of whether dose alteration is indicated during delivery to avoid neonatal problems such as respiratory depression.

Categorisation of drugs in pregnancy*

This categorisation applies only to recommended therapeutic doses in women in the reproductive age group. In situations such as overdose, occupational exposure and others when the recommended therapeutic dose is exceeded, it cannot be assumed that the classifications assigned to individual medicines are valid.

Category A

Drugs which have been taken by a large number of pregnant women and women of childbearing age without any proven increase in the frequency of malformations or other direct or indirect harmful effects on the fetus having been observed.

Category B1[†]

Drugs which have been taken by only a limited number of pregnant women and women of childbearing age, without an increase in the frequency of malformation or other direct or indirect harmful effects on the human fetus having been observed. Studies in animals have not shown evidence of an increased occurrence of fetal damage.

Category B2[†]

Drugs which have been taken by only a limited number of pregnant women and women of childbearing age, without an increase in the frequency of malformation or other direct or indirect harmful effects on the human fetus having been observed. Studies in animals are inadequate or may be lacking, but available data show no evidence of an increased occurrence of fetal damage.

Category B3[†]

Drugs which have been taken by only a limited number of pregnant women and women of childbearing age, without an increase in the frequency of malformation or other direct or indirect harmful effects on the human fetus having been observed. Studies in animals have shown

---

* *Medicines in Pregnancy Working Party of the Australian Drug Evaluation Committee. Prescribing medicines in pregnancy. An Australian categorisation of risk of drug use in pregnancy. 4th ed. Canberra: Commonwealth of Australia; 1999.*

† *For drugs in the B1, B2 and B3 categories, human data are lacking or inadequate and subcategorisation is therefore based on available animal data. The allocation of a B category does not imply greater safety than the C category.*

evidence of an increased occurrence of fetal damage, the significance of which is considered uncertain in humans.

Category C*

Drugs which, owing to their pharmacological effects, have caused or may be suspected of causing harmful effects on the human fetus or neonate without causing malformations. These effects may be reversible.

Category D†

Drugs which have caused, are suspected to have caused or may be expected to cause an increased incidence of human fetal malformations or irreversible damage. These drugs may also have adverse pharmacological effects.

Category X

Drugs which have such a high risk of causing permanent damage to the fetus that they should not be used in pregnancy or when there is a possibility of pregnancy.

Breastfeeding and the use of drugs

The benefits of breastfeeding are sufficiently important to recommend that breastfeeding be discontinued or discouraged only when there is substantial evidence that the drug taken by the mother will be harmful to the infant and that no therapeutic equivalent can be given. However, women who are known to be HIV-infected should be counselled not to breastfeed or to provide their milk for the nutrition of their own or other infants, except in areas where infectious diseases and malnutrition are major causes of infant mortality and where safe alternatives to breastfeeding are unavailable.

Most drugs are only excreted to a minimal extent in breast milk, and in most cases the dosage to which the infant is ultimately exposed is very low and well below the therapeutic dose level for infants. For this reason, there are few drugs that are totally contraindicated in women who are breastfeeding.

In most situations, drugs cross the placenta more efficiently than into breast milk.

---

* *Note that Category C in the Australian and Swedish categorisations of risk is a pharmacological effect category and differs from that in the US categorisation (where Category C indicates greater likelihood of risk than in B on the basis of adverse effects of any type in animal studies).*
† *Drugs in Category D are not absolutely contraindicated in pregnancy. Moreover, in some cases the D category has been assigned on the basis of suspicion.*

When considering prescribing medication (particularly longer-term) during breastfeeding, the following check list may assist in guiding the decision:

- **Woman's preference for breastfeeding**: Most women have a strong preference for breastfeeding. Inability to breastfeed can lead to a sense of failure as a mother, which may predispose to subsequent postnatal depression.
- **Nonpharmacological interventions**: If such an intervention is available and likely to be successful, it may allow the woman to breastfeed, at least until the period of maximum benefit to the infant has passed.
- **Risk–benefit analysis**: For the infant, there are demonstrable increases in immunocompetence (eg decreased rates of otitis media), and neurodevelopmental advantage (eg possible increased IQ in the older child). For the woman, physiological benefits of breastfeeding include decreased risk of breast cancer, better uterine involution and more delayed ovulation.
- **Education, documentation and communication**: The discussion regarding risks and benefits with the mother and her partner should be properly documented in the patient's notes. Other providers involved in postnatal management should be informed of medication changes.

The main consideration overall is that unless there is significant risk to the infant from necessary maternal medication, breastfeeding should be continued.

Table 19. Drug use in pregnancy and breastfeeding

Drug	Pregnancy category	Breastfeeding
aciclovir	B3	compatible
adrenaline	A	compatible
amoxycillin	A	compatible; may cause diarrhoea in infant
amoxycillin+clavulanate	B1	caution, no data for clavulanate; may cause diarrhoea in infant
amphotericin (oral)	B2	compatible
ampicillin	A	compatible; may cause diarrhoea in infant
articaine with adrenaline	B3	caution, insufficient data

continued next page

Table 19. Drug use in pregnancy and breastfeeding (cont.)

Drug	Pregnancy category	Breastfeeding
aspirin	C	compatible if occasional doses; avoid long-term therapy if possible, particularly in neonatal period
azathioprine	D	caution; monitor infant's immune function
azithromycin	B1	compatible; may cause diarrhoea in infant
beclomethasone dipropionate	B3	compatible
benzydamine	B2	compatible
benzylpenicillin	A	compatible; may cause diarrhoea in infant
betamethasone (topical)	A	compatible
bifonazole	B3	compatible
bupivacaine with adrenaline	A	compatible
casein phosphopeptide stabilised amorphous calcium phosphate	unlisted	compatible
cephalexin	A	compatible; may cause diarrhoea in infant
cephazolin	B1	compatible; may cause diarrhoea in infant
chlorhexidine	A	compatible
clarithromycin	B3	compatible; may cause diarrhoea in infant
clindamycin	A	compatible; may cause diarrhoea in infant
clotrimazole	A	compatible
codeine	A	compatible in occasional doses
cyclosporin	C	compatible; suggest occasional monitoring of cyclosporin blood levels in infant
dexamethasone	A	compatible

continued next page

Table 19. Drug use in pregnancy and breastfeeding (cont.)

Drug	Pregnancy category	Breastfeeding
diazepam	C	compatible in single doses—caution with long-term use; if used in latter situation, monitor infant for drowsiness
dicloxacillin	B2	compatible; may cause diarrhoea in infant
doxycycline	D*	compatible for short courses (7 to 10 days) if alternative drug not appropriate; may cause diarrhoea in infant
doxylamine	A	compatible; monitor infant for irritability and sleep disturbances
econazole	A	compatible
erythromycin	A	compatible; may cause diarrhoea in infant
famciclovir	B1	caution, insufficient data
flucloxacillin	B1	compatible; may cause diarrhoea in infant
fluconazole	D	compatible; use in consultation with a clinical microbiologist or infectious diseases physician
fluoride	unlisted	compatible
hydrocortisone	A	compatible
ibuprofen	C	compatible
idoxuridine (topical)	B1	caution, insufficient data
itraconazole	B3	caution, insufficient data
ketoconazole (systemic)	B3	caution, insufficient data
ketoconazole (topical)	B3	compatible
lignocaine	A	compatible
lignocaine with adrenaline	A	compatible
lincomycin	A	compatible; may cause diarrhoea in infant

continued next page

Table 19. Drug use in pregnancy and breastfeeding (cont.)

Drug	Pregnancy category	Breastfeeding
mepivacaine	A	caution, insufficient data
mepivacaine with adrenaline	A	caution, insufficient data
methylprednisolone aceponate (topical)	C	compatible
metronidazole (systemic)	B2	compatible; avoid high single-dose therapy
miconazole (topical)	A	compatible
mometasone furoate	B3	compatible
morphine	C	compatible; caution with high doses
naproxen	C	compatible[†]
nystatin	A	compatible
palifermin	B3	caution, insufficient data
paracetamol	A	compatible
phenoxymethylpenicillin	A	compatible; may cause diarrhoea in infant
povidone-iodine	unlisted, not recommended	avoid; may interfere with infant thyroid function
prednisolone	A	compatible
prednisone	A	compatible
prilocaine	A	compatible
prilocaine with adrenaline	A	compatible
prilocaine with felypressin	A	compatible
promethazine	C	compatible in single doses
roxithromycin	B1	compatible
teicoplanin	B3	caution, insufficient data
temazepam	C	compatible in single doses—caution with long-term use; if used in latter situation, monitor infant for drowsiness

continued next page

Table 19. Drug use in pregnancy and breastfeeding (cont.)

Drug	Pregnancy category	Breastfeeding
tetracycline	D*	compatible for short courses (7 to 10 days) if alternative drug not appropriate; may cause diarrhoea in infant
tinidazole	B3	caution, insufficient data
tranexamic acid	B1	compatible
triamcinolone acetonide (topical)	B3	compatible
triamcinolone acetonide, neomycin, gramicidin and nystatin	D	compatible
triclosan (topical)	unlisted	caution, insufficient data
trimeprazine	C	compatible; monitor infant for irritability and sleep disturbances
valaciclovir	B3	caution, insufficient data
vancomycin	B2	compatible
voriconazole	B3	avoid, insufficient data
zinc lozenges	unlisted	compatible

* Tetracyclines are safe for use during the first 18 weeks of pregnancy (16 weeks postconception) after which they may affect the formation of the baby's teeth and cause discolouration.
† If an NSAID is required in a breastfeeding patient, ibuprofen is preferred.

Abbreviations and acronyms

ADA	Australian Dental Association
AIDS	acquired immunodeficiency syndrome
amoxy/ampicillin	amoxycillin or ampicillin
BGL	blood glucose level
COPD	chronic obstructive pulmonary disease
COX	cyclo-oxygenase
CPP-ACP	casein phosphopeptide stabilised amorphous calcium phosphate
CPR	cardiopulmonary resuscitation
CYP	cytochrome P450
HIV	human immunodeficiency virus
ICU	intensive care unit
IgE	immunoglobulin E
IM	intramuscular(ly)
INR	international normalised ratio
IV	intravenous(ly)
MAOI	monoamine oxidase inhibitor
NSAID	nonsteroidal anti-inflammatory drug
OSA	obstructive sleep apnoea
PBS	Pharmaceutical Benefits Schedule
ppm	parts per million
SSRI	selective serotonin reuptake inhibitor
TCA	tricyclic antidepressant
TGL	Therapeutic Guidelines Limited
w/v	weight/volume

Glossary

The following definitions refer to the terms used in *Therapeutic Guidelines: Oral and Dental*. They may differ from definitions used in other publications.

addiction	a behavioural pattern of overwhelming involvement with the use of the drug and its procurement, and a high tendency to recidivism
agonist	a drug that stimulates activity at a cell receptor that is normally stimulated by naturally occurring substances
alveolar osteitis	a localised painful osteitis of an extraction socket following premature lysis of the blood clot
amalgam	a specific alloy used in dental restorations
anaesthesia	the loss of sensation in general (including pain)
analgesia	the removal of pain sensation
anaphylactic	pertaining to anaphylaxis
anaphylactoid	resembling anaphylaxis
anaphylaxis	an emergency condition resulting from an immediate allergic (IgE-mediated) response to a substance to which the body has become intensely sensitised
angioedema	acute oedema of the subcutaneous or submucosal tissues
angiotensin converting enzyme (ACE) inhibitors	a group of drugs used to treat cardiovascular disease; examples are captopril, enalapril, fosinopril, lisinopril, perindopril, quinapril, ramipril and trandolapril

angiotensin II receptor antagonists	a group of drugs that competitively block the binding of angiotensin to type I angiotensin II receptors. They are used to treat cardiovascular disease. Examples are candesartan, eprosartan, irbesartan, losartan and telmisartan
antagonist	a drug that binds to a cell receptor and so blocks the action of other substances that would otherwise stimulate the receptor
anticholinergic	a drug that inhibits the action of acetylcholine and so blocks the passage of impulses through the parasympathetic nervous system. Adverse effects of these drugs include dry mouth, thirst, increased heart rate, blurred vision, increased intraocular pressure, constipation, and urinary retention
anticoagulant	a drug that prevents or reduces clotting of blood; examples are heparin and warfarin
antidepressant	a drug that decreases the symptoms of depression; examples are tricyclics (amitriptyline, doxepin, dothiepin, nortriptyline, trimipramine), selective serotonin reuptake inhibitors (SSRIs) (citalopram, fluoxetine, fluvoxamine, paroxetine, sertraline), mianserin, nefazodone, reboxetine, venlafaxine, and monoamine oxidase inhibitors (MAOIs) (phenelzine, moclobemide, tranylcypromine)
antiepileptic	a drug used in the management of seizures; examples are carbamazepine, ethosuximide, phenobarbitone, phenytoin, primidone, sodium valproate, gabapentin, lamotrigine, tiagabine, topiramate and vigabatrin
antihistamine	a drug that inhibits the action of histamine in the body by blocking the receptors for histamine. There are two types of histamine receptors—H_1 and H_2. Stimulation of H_1 receptors may produce allergic reactions such as hay fever and itch; antihistamines that block H_1 receptors include dexchlorpheniramine, pheniramine, methdilazine, promethazine, trimeprazine, cetirizine, azatadine, cyproheptadine, fexofenadine and loratadine. Stimulation of H_2 receptors, which are found mainly in the stomach, causes acid secretion; H_2-receptor antagonists include cimetidine, famotidine, nizatidine and ranitidine

antiparkinsonian drugs	drugs used to treat Parkinson's disease, and to reduce some extrapyramidal effects caused by antipsychotic drugs; they include benztropine, benzhexol, biperiden and orphenadrine
antiplatelet drugs	drugs that inhibit platelet aggregation, or inhibit platelet function in some other manner; examples are aspirin, clopidogrel, ticlopidine and abciximab
antipsychotic drugs	drugs used in the treatment of psychoses; they include amisulpride, aripiprazole, chlorpromazine, clozapine, droperidol, flupenthixol, fluphenazine, haloperidol, olanzapine, pericyazine, pimozide, quetiapine, risperidone, thioridazine, trifluoperazine, ziprasidone and zuclopenthixol
antiretroviral drugs	drugs used in the treatment of AIDS; they include nucleoside/nucleotide reverse transcriptase inhibitors (eg abacavir, lamivudine, zidovudine), non-nucleoside reverse transcriptase inhibitors (eg efavirenz, nevirapine), protease inhibitors (eg indinavir, ritonavir) and HIV-entry inhibitors (eg enfuvirtide)
antiseptic	a substance that inhibits the growth and development of microorganisms by physical or chemical means
anxiolytic	a drug used to reduce anxiety; examples are benzodiazepines (eg clonazepam, diazepam, midazolam, lorazepam, alprazolam)
apical periodontitis	inflammation of the periodontal ligament and bone surrounding the apex or end of a tooth root
apicoectomy	resection of the apex of a tooth root (usually performed in conjunction with a curettage of the periapical tissues and the placement of a retrograde root filling)
asthenia	weakness, loss of strength
atrial fibrillation	a cardiac arrhythmia with a rapid and irregular heart rate
azoles	drugs used to treat fungal infections; examples are bifonazole, clotrimazole, econazole, fluconazole, itraconazole, ketoconazole, miconazole, posaconazole and voriconazole

benzodiazepines	the most commonly prescribed anxiolytic and sedative drugs; they also have antiepileptic, muscle relaxant and memory impairing actions. Examples are clonazepam, diazepam, midazolam, lorazepam and alprazolam
beta lactam	a class of antibiotics. They include carbapenems, cephalosporins, monobactams and penicillins
$beta_2$ agonists	drugs that relax smooth muscle of the airway resulting in bronchodilation. They are used in asthma and other respiratory conditions. Examples are salbutamol, terbutaline, eformoterol and salmeterol
beta-blocking drugs	a group of drugs that competitively antagonise beta adrenoceptors and are used in the treatment of some cardiovascular disease; examples are atenolol, bisoprolol, carvedilol, esmolol, labetalol, metoprolol, oxprenolol, pindolol, propranolol and sotalol
biofilm	a community of microorganisms adhering in a thin layer to a surface. The community has a collective physiology and works together
bisphosphonates	drugs that slow bone loss by reducing bone resorption; examples are alendronate, disodium pamidronate, etidronate, risedronate, sodium clodronate, tiludronate and zoledronic acid
bridge	a dental prosthesis used to replace one or more missing teeth and which is cemented on to the adjacent teeth
bronchodilator	a drug that relaxes and dilates the bronchial passageways and improves the passage of air into the lungs; examples are salbutamol, terbutaline, eformoterol, salmeterol, ipratropium and tiotropium
calculus (dental)	hard deposit of mineralised material adhering to teeth
caries	commonly used term for tooth decay
cementum	hard connective tissue covering the root of a tooth

cephalosporins	one group of beta-lactam antibiotics; examples are cephalexin, cephalothin, cephazolin, cefuroxime, cefaclor, cefoxitin, cefotaxime, ceftriaxone, ceftazidime and cefepime
cholinergic	releasing or activated by acetylcholine or a related compound
cholinesterase inhibitors	drugs used in the treatment of mild to moderately severe dementia; examples are donepezil, galantamine and rivastigmine
clastic	a general term used for cells that resorb hard tissue such as bone, cementum and dentine
CMI (consumer medicines information) leaflets	especially written leaflets for consumers (patients) that provide information about medicines and how to use them
combination therapy	therapy that uses two or more drugs in the treatment of a single disease
continuous positive airway pressure (CPAP)	a treatment that may be required for patients with moderate to severe obstructive sleep apnoea. It works by pneumatically splinting the upper airway, preventing its closure during sleep. It is achieved by machines specifically designed to blow air via a flexible hose into a close-fitting nasal mask, which is worn during sleep
coronal	pertaining to the clinical crown of a tooth
corticosteroids	steroid hormones produced by the adrenal cortex, or their synthetic equivalents. They can be used orally, topically, systemically, inta-articularly and by inhalation. Inhaled corticosteroids include beclomethasone dipropionate, budesonide and fluticasone propionate; oral corticosteroids are prednisolone and prednisone; parenteral corticosteroids include dexamethasone, hydrocortisone and methylprednisolone
cytochrome P450 (CYP) enzymes	a group of enzymes that control the concentrations of many endogenous substances and drugs
dentine	the part of the tooth beneath enamel and cementum
dentifrice	toothpaste

dependence, physical	the need for a drug such that withdrawal symptoms occur when the drug is discontinued
diaphoresis	sweating
differential diagnosis	the list of possible diagnoses formed during the process of systematically determining what disease or condition is present
directed treatment	specific therapy that is based on culture and susceptibility test results
diuretic	a drug that increases the excretion of urine; examples are the thiazide diuretics (eg hydrochlorothiazide), frusemide, bumetanide, ethacrynic acid, spironolactone, amiloride and triamterene
dry socket	common name for alveolar osteitis
empirical treatment	therapy that is based on experience (eg of known common pathogens in the condition and their current resistance patterns)
enamel	hard calcified tissue covering the dentine of the crown of a tooth
endodontics / endodontic treatment	root canal treatment; a process where the dental pulp and/or infected debris is removed from the tooth and its root canal system which is then cleaned, disinfected and then filled
eugenol	a liquid phenol—$C_{10}H_{12}O_2$—contained in certain essential oils (eg cloves), used in some dental materials as a therapeutic agent to reduce pulp inflammation and to arrest dental caries
extrapyramidal effects	motor movements not related to the pyramidal tract. These include akathisia (motor restlessness), dystonias (twisting and contractions of muscle groups), pseudoparkinsonism (stiffness, shuffling, tremors, motor rigidity), and tardive dyskinesia (involuntary irregular muscle movements, usually in the face)
fluorapatite	$Ca_{10}(PO_4)_6F_2$—a crystal formed when fluoride is incorporated into tooth enamel during formation of the tooth

fluorhydroxyapatite	$Ca_{10}(PO_4)_6(OH)F$—a crystal formed when fluoride is incorporated into tooth enamel during formation of the tooth
fluoride	a compound containing the element fluorine. It reduces the rate of demineralisation of teeth and enhances mineral uptake
fluorosis (dental)	an irreversible condition caused by excessive ingestion of fluoride during the tooth-forming years. Excess fluoride causes dental fluorosis by damaging the enamel-forming cells. The damage to these cells results in a mineralisation disorder of the teeth, whereby the porosity of the subsurface enamel is increased. The teeth may have white spots, various discolourations and/or mottling of the enamel
gingiva	commonly known as the gum tissue, this soft tissue encircles the necks of erupted teeth and covers the crowns of unerupted teeth
glycopeptides	a group of antibiotics; examples are teicoplanin and vancomycin
Gram stain	a method of differentiating bacteria into two large groups (Gram-positive and Gram-negative) based on the chemical and physical properties of their cell walls
half-life (of a drug)	the time required for half the quantity of a drug to be metabolised or eliminated by normal processes
$histamine_2$ receptor	one of the two types of histamine receptors. Drugs that block H_2 receptors include cimetidine, famotidine, nizatidine and ranitidine
hydrophilic	readily absorbing or dissolving in water
hydroxyapatite	$Ca_{10}(PO_4)_6(OH)_2$—part of the structure of tooth enamel
hyphae	thread-like structure in the mycelium of a fungus
hypnotics	drugs that induce sleep; examples are nitrazepam, oxazepam, temazepam, zolpidem and zopiclone
hypoglycaemia	low level of glucose in the blood

hypoglycaemic drugs	drugs used in the treatment of diabetes to lower the blood glucose level; examples are glibenclamide, gliclazide, glimepiride, glipizide, metformin, pioglitazone, repaglinide and rosiglitazone
intraligamentous/ intraligamentary local anaesthetic	a technique for local anaesthesia of the teeth where the anaesthetic solution is injected under pressure into the periodontal ligament of the tooth to be treated
immunocompromised	incapable of developing a normal immune response, usually as a result of disease, malnutrition, or immunosuppressive therapy
immunodeficiency	deficiency in the immune response
immunoglobulin E (IgE)	one of the five major classes of immunoglobulins that function as antibodies; other classes are IgA, IgD, IgG and IgM
impacted tooth	an unerupted or partially erupted tooth that is positioned against another structure so that complete eruption is unlikely
implant, dental	a device designed to be placed surgically into the oral tissues to provide a base for a dental prosthesis; it is usually made of titanium
incidence	the number of new cases occurring in a population within a specific time period
infiltration	a technique for local anaesthesia where the injection is given adjacent to the location where the effect of the anaesthetic is required
intradental	within a tooth; typically used to describe the placement of a drug or dental material within a cavity or in the root canal system
intraosseous local anaesthetic	a technique for local anaesthesia of the teeth where a small opening is made through the cortical plate of the bone near the tooth to be treated, and the local anaesthetic solution is injected directly into the underlying cancellous bone
keratin	a protein that is a major component of epidermis, nails and hair

ketoacidosis	acidosis with an accumulation of ketone bodies; occurs primarily in patients with diabetes, where it is usually accompanied by dehydration, hyperglycaemia, and insulin deficiency
leukoplakia	a white patch or plaque that cannot be removed and cannot be characterised clinically (or histologically) as any other pathology
lincosamides	a class of antibiotics; examples are clindamycin and lincomycin
lipophilic	having an affinity for lipids
macrolides	a class of antibiotics; examples are azithromycin, clarithromycin, erythromycin and roxithromycin
management	the act, art and manner of handling a situation; it includes treatment, but also includes the overall handling of the patient and their problems in a sensitive manner
mandibular advancement splint	a device usually made from acrylic and worn on the teeth to hold the mandibular teeth in a protruded position in order to keep the airway open; it can be used to treat sleep apnoea and to prevent snoring
methaemoglobin	a brown pigment formed from haemoglobin by oxidisation of the ferrous to the ferric state. A small amount is present normally in the blood. It does not reversibly carry oxygen (unlike haemoglobin)
methaemoglobinaemia	excessive amounts of methaemoglobin in the blood, which results in decreased oxygen to the tissues
miosis	contraction of the pupil of the eye
monoamine oxidase inhibitors (MAOIs)	a class of antidepressant drugs; examples are phenelzine, moclobemide and tranylcypromine
mu-receptors	one of the classes of binding sites for opioid drugs (others are delta and kappa). The classes are differentiated on the basis of their binding characteristics and selective sensitivities to different opioids
muscarinic receptors	cholinergic receptors that are stimulated by muscarine and blocked by atropine

narcotic	opioid
neuropathic pain	pain initiated or caused by a primary lesion or dysfunction in the nervous system. Peripheral neuropathic pain occurs when the lesion or dysfunction affects the peripheral nervous system
nitroimidazoles	a class of antibiotics; examples are metronidazole and tinidazole
nociceptive pain	pain arising from stimulation of nociceptors by noxious stimuli
nociceptor	a receptor preferentially sensitive to a noxious stimulus or to a stimulus which would become noxious if prolonged
occlusion	the way the teeth bite together
occlusal splint	a device usually made from acrylic and worn on the teeth to distribute the load placed on the teeth during biting, grinding and clenching; it can be used to treat some temporomandibular dysfunction conditions and to prevent wearing of the teeth
odontogenic	tooth-related
operculum	loose flap of gingival or mucosal tissue overlying a partially erupted tooth
opioid	agonists and partial agonists with morphine-like activity, including naturally-occurring and synthetic compounds; examples are alfentanil, buprenorphine, codeine, dextromoramide, dextropropoxyphene, fentanyl, hydromorphone, methadone, morphine, oxycodone, pethidine, remifentanil, sufentanil and tramadol
osteonecrosis	necrosis of bone
osteoradionecrosis	necrosis of bone following radiation therapy
parasympathomimetic	a drug that produces effects similar to those of stimulation of the parasympathetic nerve supply
parenteral	by other than the gastrointestinal system (eg subcutaneous, intramuscular, intravenous, intradental, intra-articular)

penicillins	a group of beta-lactam antibiotics; examples are amoxycillin, ampicillin, benzathine penicillin, benzylpenicillin, dicloxacillin, flucloxacillin, methicillin, phenoxymethylpenicillin, piperacillin, procaine penicillin, and ticarcillin
periodic acid–Schiff reaction	a laboratory test using periodic acid and Schiff reagent; it is used in the diagnosis of some systemic diseases and fungal infections
periodontal	pertaining to the supporting and surrounding tissues of the teeth—the gingivae, the periodontal ligament, the cementum and the alveolar bone
periodontal ligament	the fibrous connective tissue that surrounds the root of a tooth, attaching it to the bone
periodontitis	inflammation of the supporting structures of the teeth—the periodontal ligament, cementum and alveolar bone; common name for periodontal disease
pH	a means of expressing acidity and alkalinity. The pH scale ranges from 0 to 14, with 7 being neutral; numbers increase with increasing alkalinity, and decrease with increasing acidity
pKa	the negative logarithm of the equilibrium constant (Ka) of the acid-base reaction of a compound; more negative pKa values correspond to stronger acids and more positive pKa values correspond to weaker acids
plaque	a complex biofilm of microorganisms and their by-products that builds up on the teeth
polydipsia	chronic excessive thirst and fluid intake
polyenes	a group of antibiotics; examples are amphotericin and nystatin
polyuria	large amount of urine excretion
prescription-only drug	a drug that can only be obtained with a prescription; it cannot be bought 'over the counter'
prevalence	the proportion of a population affected at a particular time

proton pump inhibitors	a group of drugs that suppress gastric acid secretion; examples are omeprazole, esomeprazole, lansoprazole, pantoprazole and rabeprazole
provisional diagnosis	the clinician's initial diagnosis based on the patient's history and information available up to that point in time; further diagnostic information and test results are still required before a definitive diagnosis can be made; in some situations, the response to initial treatment may need to be assessed before the provisional diagnosis can be considered as being correct or incorrect
psychogenic disorders	syndromes in which the patient presents with symptoms that predominantly suggest an organic disorder, but the medical history, physical examination and investigations do not demonstrate any organic disease that could explain the symptoms
psychostimulants	drugs that stimulate the brain. They include the amphetamines (eg dexamphetamine), methylphenidate, modafinil, cocaine, ecstasy and related substances
pulpitis	inflammation of the dental pulp; this inflammation may be acute or chronic, reversible or irreversible
radicular	pertaining to the root
regional block	a local anaesthetic technique where the anaesthetic solution is injected adjacent to the target nerve, but at a distance proximal to the site where the anaesthesia is required
restoration	commonly known as a filling or a crown; when a dental material has been used to restore, rebuild or replace lost tooth structure; various materials can be used, including metal alloys, resins, glass ionomers, and porcelains
retrognathia	abnormality of craniofacial anatomy, with posterior positioning of the jaw relative to the facial skeleton

Reye's syndrome	a rare, serious, potentially fatal condition that affects children; it most often occurs following a viral infection
root planing	a procedure to remove microbial flora, plaque, bacterial toxins, calculus and affected cementum or dentine on the root surfaces and in a periodontal pocket
rubber dam	a sheet of rubber that is placed over the teeth to isolate the operating field while doing procedures to the teeth
scaling	a procedure to remove plaque and calculus from teeth
selective serotonin reuptake inhibitors (SSRIs)	one class of antidepressant drugs; examples are citalopram, fluoxetine, fluvoxamine, paroxetine and sertraline
somatoform	a mental disorder presenting with physical symptoms
statins	hydroxymethylglutaryl coenzyme A reductase inhibitors, which reduce concentrations of total cholesterol and low-density lipoprotein cholesterol and to a lesser extent triglycerides; examples are atorvastatin, fluvastatin, pravastatin and simvastatin
T cells	the group of lymphocytes primarily responsible for cell-mediated immunity
temporise	to place a temporary restoration in a tooth
third molar model	a clinical model developed following studies of third molar surgery. It is useful for evaluating the efficacy of analgesics, anti-inflammatory drugs, local anaesthetic solutions and surgical techniques
tolerance	a physical state whereby, after repeated administration, a given dose of drug produces a decreased effect, or increasingly larger doses must be taken to obtain the effects observed with the original dose
treatment	a systematic course of medical or surgical care; a part of management

tricyclic antidepressants (TCAs)	a class of antidepressant drugs; examples are amitriptyline, clomipramine, dothiepin, doxepin, imipramine, nortriptyline and trimipramine
trismus	restricted ability to open the mouth
urticaria	transient erythematous raised oedematous wheals
viral load	the number of copies of RNA of a given virus per millilitre of blood. Monitoring viral load is important in managing chronic viral infections (eg HIV) and in immunocompromised patients
xerostomia	dry mouth

Index

Page numbers followed by 'b' refer to boxes, by 'f' to figures, by 'p' to photos, and by 't' to tables.

A

abbreviations	203
aciclovir	
clinical pharmacology	28
pregnancy and breastfeeding	
risk categorisation	197t
therapeutic use	
herpes labialis	116
acronyms	203
Acts (legislation) relating to drugs and prescriptions	11
acute myocardial infarction	168
management	169b
acute necrotising ulcerative gingivitis	99
with HIV	100
Acute odontogenic infections	127–34
acute ulcerative gingivitis	99
with HIV	100
addiction	57
Addison's disease	74
Addisonian crisis	74, 179
management	179b
adrenal crisis	74, 179
management	179b
adrenal disorders	74
Addisonian crisis	74
Addison's disease	74
adrenal crisis	74
adrenal suppression	74
adrenal suppression	74
adrenaline	
clinical pharmacology	52
properties and strengths in local anaesthetics	50t
interactions	53
pregnancy and breastfeeding	
risk categorisation	197t
therapeutic use	
anaphylactic and anaphylactoid reactions	183, 184b, 186b

airway obstruction	174
management	174b
signs	174t
alcohol in mouthwashes	58
alkalosis, gaseous	170
management	171b
allergic reactions	
(see also allergies)	181
anaphylactic and anaphylactoid	182
management	183b, 184b
angioedema	182
urticaria	181
management	182b
allergies (see also allergic reactions)	179–87
causes	180
antibiotic	15, 180
penicillin	17
food	181
latex	180
local anaesthetics	180
types of allergic reactions	181
alveolar osteitis	134
amalgam, hypersensitivity to	
as cause of lichen planus	110
amifostine	
therapeutic use	
mucositis	122
amoxycillin	
adverse effects	21, 22
clinical pharmacology	21, 22
interactions	21, 23
precautions	21
pregnancy and breastfeeding	
risk categorisation	197t
therapeutic use	
dentoalveolar surgery	
infection following	133
prophylaxis for	141
endocarditis prophylaxis	137

amoxycillin (cont.)
  therapeutic use (cont.)
    odontogenic infections
        129, 130, 131
    periodontal abscess   101
amoxycillin + clavulanate
  adverse effects   21, 22, 23
  clinical pharmacology   21, 22, 23
  interactions   21
  precautions   21
  pregnancy and breastfeeding
    risk categorisation   197t
  therapeutic use
    odontogenic infections   130
amphotericin
  adverse effects   28
  clinical pharmacology   28
  pregnancy and breastfeeding
    risk categorisation   197t
  therapeutic use
    candidosis   119
ampicillin
  pregnancy and breastfeeding
    risk categorisation   197t
ampicillin (see also amoxycillin)
  adverse effects   21, 22
  clinical pharmacology   21, 22
  interactions   21, 23
  precautions   21
  therapeutic use
    odontogenic infections   131
anaesthesia, local
    see local anaesthesia
anaesthetics, local
    see local anaesthetics
analgesics   29–36
  (see also individual drugs and local anaesthetics)
  clinical pharmacology   29
  principles of use   146
  use in dentistry   147
anaphylactic reactions   182
  management   183b, 184b
anaphylactoid reactions   182
  management   183b, 184b
angina
  dental issues in patients with   65
  management   168b
angioedema   182
antibiotic hypersensitivity   15, 180
antibiotic prophylaxis   135–43
    see prophylaxis (antibiotic)
antibiotic-associated diarrhoea   17

antibiotics   13–29
  (see also individual groups and drugs)
  administration methods   20
  choice of   18
  clinical pharmacology   21
  principles of use   13, 14b
  problems with   15
    contraceptives and   18
    diarrhoea associated with   17
    hypersensitivity (allergy)   15, 180
    pseudomembranous colitis
      associated with   17
    resistance of   15
  used in dentistry   16t
anticoagulants
  problems with dental treatment   62
antifungal drugs
  (see also individual drugs)
  examples of   16t
antihistamines   55
  adverse effects   56
  xerostomia   122
antimicrobials   see antibiotics
antiplatelet drugs
  problems with dental treatment   62
antiviral drugs
  (see also individual drugs)
  clinical pharmacology   28
  examples of   17t
ANUG   see acute ulcerative gingivitis
aphthous ulcers   114
articaine
  adverse effects
    local   158
    systemic   47, 52
  clinical pharmacology   52
    properties and maximum doses   51t
  pregnancy and breastfeeding
    risk categorisation   197t
  therapeutic use
    local anaesthesia   158
artificial joint
  prevention of infection   140
    dental treatment and   142b
aspirin
  adverse effects   30, 31t
    Reye's syndrome   31
    risk factors for gastrointestinal   32t
  clinical pharmacology   31
    third molar model   154b
  interactions   30
  precautions   30, 62

aspirin (cont.)
- precautions (cont.)
  - dental management of patients taking — 63
- pregnancy and breastfeeding risk categorisation — 198t
- principles of use — 29
- therapeutic use
  - myocardial infarction — 169b
  - pain, post-treatment (adults) — 150

asthma
- acute attack — 171
- assessment — 172t
- dental issues in patients with — 67
- management — 173b

AUG   see acute ulcerative gingivitis

azathioprine
- pregnancy and breastfeeding risk categorisation — 198t

azithromycin
- adverse effects — 25
- clinical pharmacology — 25
- interactions — 26
- pregnancy and breastfeeding risk categorisation — 198t

azoles (see also individual drugs)
- adverse effects — 28
- clinical pharmacology — 27
- examples of — 16t
- interactions — 28

B

bacteraemia
- bleeding and — 135
- dental procedures and risk of — 137t
- relationship between dental procedure and bacteraemia — 139f

Basic life support flow chart — 187f

beclomethasone dipropionate
- adverse effects — 42
- clinical pharmacology
  - potency — 40t
- pregnancy and breastfeeding risk categorisation — 198t
- principles of use — 38
- therapeutic use — 40t
  - aphthous ulcers — 115
  - lichen planus — 111

benzodiazepines — 53
- adverse effects — 54
- clinical pharmacology — 53
- contraindications — 54
- precautions — 54

benzydamine
(see also mouthwashes)
- adverse effects — 60
- clinical pharmacology — 60
- pregnancy and breastfeeding risk categorisation — 198t
- therapeutic use
  - herpes gingivostomatitis — 116
  - mucositis — 123t
  - viral ulcers — 116
  - xerostomia — 123t

benzylpenicillin
- adverse effects — 21, 22
- clinical pharmacology — 21, 22
- interactions — 21
- precautions — 21
- pregnancy and breastfeeding risk categorisation — 198t
- therapeutic use
  - dentoalveolar surgery prophylaxis for — 141
  - odontogenic infections — 131

beta lactams
(see also individual drugs)
- adverse effects — 21
- clinical pharmacology — 21
- examples of — 16t
- interactions — 21
- precautions — 21

betamethasone
- adverse effects — 42
- clinical pharmacology
  - potency — 40t
- pregnancy and breastfeeding risk categorisation — 198t
- principles of use — 38
- therapeutic use — 40t
  - aphthous ulcers — 115
  - lichen planus — 110

bifonazole
- adverse effects — 28
- clinical pharmacology — 27
- interactions — 28
- pregnancy and breastfeeding risk categorisation — 198t

bisphosphonates
- adverse effects
  - osteonecrosis of the jaws — 76
- bone surgery and — 78
- dental issues in patients taking — 76
  - bone surgery — 78
  - extractions — 78
  - history-taking — 76b
- extractions and — 78

bisphosphonates (cont.)
  individual drugs — 76b
  requirements before initiating treatment — 78
  therapeutic use
    bone disease — 75
    osteoporosis — 75
black hairy tongue — 111
bleeding in patients taking anticoagulants
  risk with surgery — 62
blood glucose levels — 71
breastfeeding and drugs — 196
  risk categorisation of individual drugs — 197t
bupivacaine
  adverse effects
    local — 158
    systemic — 47
  clinical pharmacology — 52
    properties and maximum doses — 51t
  pregnancy and breastfeeding
    risk categorisation — 198t
  therapeutic use
    local anaesthesia — 52
    trigeminal neuralgia — 82

C

cancer of the head and neck
  dental issues in patients with — 84
candidiasis *see* candidosis
candidosis — 118
  management — 119
  predisposing factors — 119
carbapenems
  examples of — 16t
cardiac arrest — 170
  management — 170b
cardiac conditions with risk for endocarditis — 136t
cardiomyopathy
  dental issues in patients with — 67
cardiovascular conditions — 61
  anticoagulant and antiplatelet drugs — 62
  cardiomyopathy — 67
  coronary ischaemic disease — 65
  heart failure — 66
  hypertension — 63
  prevention of — 62
cardiovascular emergencies — 166
  cardiac arrest — 170
  coronary ischaemic disease — 166
  syncope — 166

caries — 91–6
  modifying factors — 92
  pathophysiology — 91
  stages of (schematic diagram) — 128f
  treatment — 92
  xerostomia and — 122
casein phosphopeptide stabilised amorphous calcium phosphate
  clinical pharmacology — 94
  pregnancy and breastfeeding
    risk categorisation — 198t
  therapeutic use
    caries prevention — 95t
categorisation of drugs in pregnancy — 195
  individual drugs — 197–201t
cephalexin
  adverse effects — 21, 24
  clinical pharmacology — 21, 23
  interactions — 21, 24
  precautions — 21
  pregnancy and breastfeeding
    risk categorisation — 198t
  therapeutic use
    endocarditis prophylaxis — 139
cephalosporins
  (*see also individual drugs*)
  adverse effects — 21, 24
  clinical pharmacology — 21, 23
  examples of — 16t
  interactions — 21, 24
  precautions — 21
cephazolin
  adverse effects — 21, 24
  clinical pharmacology — 21, 23
  interactions — 21, 24
  precautions — 21
  pregnancy and breastfeeding
    risk categorisation — 198t
  therapeutic use
    odontogenic infections — 131
cheilitis, angular — 120
chemotherapy
  adverse effects
    mucositis — 121
  dental issues in patients having — 85
chlorhexidine
  (*see also* mouthwashes)
  adverse effects — 59
    hairy tongue — 111
  clinical pharmacology — 59, 94
  interactions — 94
  pregnancy and breastfeeding
    risk categorisation — 198t

chlorhexidine (cont.)
  therapeutic use
    acute ulcerative gingivitis — 100
    caries prevention — 94, 95t
    gingivitis — 98
      acute ulcerative gingivitis — 100
    halitosis — 105
    herpes gingivostomatitis — 116
    mucositis — 123t
    viral ulcers — 116
    xerostomia — 123t
cholinesterase, atypical — 46
chronic obstructive pulmonary disease
  dental issues in patients with — 69
clarithromycin
  adverse effects — 25
  clinical pharmacology — 25
  interactions — 26
  pregnancy and breastfeeding
    risk categorisation — 198t
clavulanate
      see amoxycillin+clavulanate
clindamycin
  adverse effects — 25
  clinical pharmacology — 25
  pregnancy and breastfeeding
    risk categorisation — 198t
  therapeutic use
    dentoalveolar procedures
      infection following — 133
      prophylaxis for — 141
    endocarditis prophylaxis — 138
    odontogenic infections — 129, 130, 131
    periodontal abscess — 101
clotrimazole
  adverse effects — 28
  clinical pharmacology — 27
  interactions — 28
  pregnancy and breastfeeding
    risk categorisation — 198t
codeine
  adverse effects — 34, 25t
  clinical pharmacology — 36
    third molar model — 154b
  interactions — 36
  precautions — 36
  pregnancy and breastfeeding
    risk categorisation — 198t
  principles of use — 146
  therapeutic use
    pain, post-treatment (adult) — 150
consent and sedation — 162

contact dermatitis
  latex allergy — 180
contraceptives (oral) and antibiotics — 18
coronary ischaemic disease — 65
  dental issues in patients with — 65
  emergencies — 166
corticosteroids — 36–45
  (see also individual drugs)
  intradermal — 37
  intralesional
    therapeutic use
      aphthous ulcers — 115
      lichen planus — 111
  systemic — 44
    adverse effects — 45
      adrenal crisis — 74
      adrenal suppression — 74
    dosing
      before dental procedures — 75
    therapeutic use
      Addisonian (adrenal) crisis — 179
      anaphylactic and anaphylactoid reactions — 186b
      aphthous ulcers — 115
      lichen planus — 111
  topical — 38–43
    adverse effects — 42
    individual — 40t
    principles of use — 38
    therapeutic use
      aphthous ulcers — 115
      lichen planus — 110
CPP-ACP
      see casein phosphopeptide stabilised amorphous calcium phosphate
cyclosporin
  pregnancy and breastfeeding
    risk categorisation — 198t

D

decay (tooth) — see caries
Dental caries — 91–6
dental implants
  infection following — 143
dental infections
      see odontogenic infections
Dental management of patients taking medications — 61–90
dental pain — see pain management
dental procedures
      see procedures (dental)
dentoalveolar procedures
      see procedures (dental)

dependence (drug)	57
dexamethasone	
adverse effects	45
clinical pharmacology	45
pregnancy and breastfeeding	
risk categorisation	198t
therapeutic use	
anaphylactic and anaphylactoid reactions	186b
diabetes	
dental issues in patients with	70
diabetic control	71
healing problems	72
infections	71
emergencies	177
hypoglycaemia	177
ketoacidosis	178
routine dental treatment and	73b
diabetic ketoacidosis	178
management	179b
diagnosis, principles of	1–4
diarrhoea, antibiotic-associated	17
diazepam	
adverse effects	54
clinical pharmacology	54
contraindications	54
interactions	55
precautions	54, 55
pregnancy and breastfeeding	
risk categorisation	199t
therapeutic use	
sedation	162
dicloxacillin	
adverse effects	21, 22
clinical pharmacology	21, 22
interactions	21
precautions	21
pregnancy and breastfeeding	
risk categorisation	199t
directed therapy (definition)	19
discolouration of teeth with tetracyclines	26
documentation	
of diagnosis in patient's history	3b
doxycycline	
adverse effects	26
children and	26
clinical pharmacology	26
interactions	27
precautions	26
pregnancy and breastfeeding	26
risk categorisation	199t
doxylamine	
adverse effects	56

doxylamine (cont.)	
clinical pharmacology	56
pregnancy and breastfeeding	
risk categorisation	199t
therapeutic use	
pain, post-treatment (adults)	150
drug information, sources of	10
drug prescribing	7
(see also prescriptions and prescription-writing)	
drugs and sport	191
drugs during pregnancy and breastfeeding	193
drugs required for emergencies	188
dry socket	134
dysaesthesia	
local anaesthesia causing	159

E

econazole	
adverse effects	28
clinical pharmacology	27
interactions	28
pregnancy and breastfeeding	
risk categorisation	199t
emergencies (medical)	165–87
drugs and equipment required	188
types	
allergies	179
anaphylactic and anaphylactoid reactions	182
cardiovascular	166
endocrine	177
neurological	176
respiratory	170
emergency drugs and equipment	188
empirical therapy (definition)	19
endocarditis prophylaxis	135
cardiac conditions and	136t
dental procedures and risk of bacteraemia	137t
endocrine conditions	70
adrenal disorders	74
diabetes	70
thyroid disorders	72
endocrine emergencies	177
Addisonian (adrenal) crisis	179
diabetic ketoacidosis	178
hypoglycaemia	177
epilepsy	
dental issues in patients with	80
emergency management	177b
equipment required for emergencies	188

erythema migrans	111
erythema multiforme	118
erythematous candidosis	118
erythromycin	
adverse effects	25
clinical pharmacology	25
interactions	26
pregnancy and breastfeeding	
risk categorisation	199t
extractions	
infection following	141
osteonecrosis of the jaws and	76
osteoradionecrosis and	85
patients taking aspirin	63
patients taking bisphosphonates	78
patients taking warfarin	63
procedure for	64b
radiotherapy and	85

F

facial nerve weakness	
dental issues in patients with	80
famciclovir	28
pregnancy and breastfeeding	
risk categorisation	199t
famotidine	
therapeutic use	
anaphylactic and anaphylactoid reactions	185b
felypressin	
adverse effects	53
clinical pharmacology	53
properties and strengths in local anaesthetics	50t
contraindications	53
flucloxacillin	
adverse effects	21, 22
clinical pharmacology	21, 22
interactions	21
precautions	21
pregnancy and breastfeeding	
risk categorisation	199t
fluconazole	
adverse effects	28
clinical pharmacology	27
interactions	28
pregnancy and breastfeeding	
risk categorisation	199t
therapeutic use	
candidosis	120
fluoride	
adverse effects	
fluorosis	93

fluoride (cont.)	
children and	93
clinical pharmacology	93
topical applications	95t
pregnancy and breastfeeding	
risk categorisation	199t
therapeutic use	
caries prevention	94, 95t
xerostomia	124
fluoride supplements	93
fluorosis	93
food allergy	181
fungal infections	118
angular cheilitis	120
candidosis	118

G

geographic tongue	111
Getting to know your drugs	13–60
gingival hyperplasia	81
gingivitis	97
acute ulcerative	99
gingivostomatitis (viral)	115
glossary	205–18
glucose levels (blood)	71
glyceryl trinitrate	
therapeutic use	
angina	168b
myocardial infarction	169b
glycopeptides	
(see also individual drugs)	
adverse effects	25
clinical pharmacology	24
examples of	16t
guanine analogues	
(see also individual drugs)	
clinical pharmacology	28
examples of	17t

H

hairy leukoplakia	112, 112p
hairy tongue	111
halimeter	104
halitosis	103–5
causes of	104b
diagnosis	104
management	103
pathophysiology	103
hand foot and mouth disease	115
head and neck cancer	
dental issues in patients with	84
heart failure	
dental issues in patients with	66

hepatitis B
dental issues in patients with 83
hepatitis C
dental issues in patients with 83
xerostomia and 122
herpangina 115
herpes gingivostomatitis 115
herpes labialis 116
history and history-taking
components of 2
documentation 3b
relating to bisphosphonates 76b
HIV
see human immunodeficiency virus
human immunodeficiency virus 84
acute ulcerative gingivitis and 100
dental issues in patients with 84
hydrocortisone (systemic)
pregnancy and breastfeeding
risk categorisation 199t
therapeutic use
Addisonian (adrenal) crisis 179b
anaphylactic and anaphylactoid
reactions 186b
hydrocortisone acetate (topical)
adverse effects 42
clinical pharmacology
potency 40t
pregnancy and breastfeeding
risk categorisation 199t
principles of use 38
therapeutic use 40t
hyperplastic candidosis 119
hypersensitivity to antibiotics 15, 180
to penicillin 17
hypertension
dental issues in patients with 63
hyperthyroidism
dental issues in patients with 73
hyperventilation syndrome 170
management 171b
hypnotics 53
hypoglycaemia 177
management 178b
hypothyroidism
dental issues in patients with 72
hypovitaminosis
as cause of mucositis 121

I

ibuprofen
administration 146
adverse effects 30, 31t
risk factors for gastrointestinal 32t

ibuprofen (cont.)
clinical pharmacology 32
interactions 30
precautions 30
pregnancy and breastfeeding
risk categorisation 199t
principles of use 29
therapeutic use
pain, post-treatment
adults 149, 150
children 151
idoxuridine
clinical pharmacology 29
pregnancy and breastfeeding
risk categorisation 199t
therapeutic use
herpes labialis 116
illnesses (medical) 61–90
implants, infection following 143
infections (tooth-related)
see odontogenic infections
infiltration anaesthesia 157
informed consent and sedation 162
inhaled objects 173
management 174b
prevention 172
intraligamentous anaesthesia 157
intraosseous anaesthesia 157
isosorbide dinitrate
therapeutic use
angina 168b
myocardial infarction 169b
itraconazole
adverse effects 28
clinical pharmacology 27
interactions 28
pregnancy and breastfeeding
risk categorisation 199t
therapeutic use
candidosis 120

J

joint prosthesis
prevention of infection 140
dental treatment and 142b

K

ketoacidosis (diabetic) 178
management 179b
ketoconazole
adverse effects 28
clinical pharmacology 27
interactions 28

ketoconazole (cont.)
   pregnancy and breastfeeding
      risk categorisation   199t

L

latex allergy   180
legislation about prescriptions
   and prescribing   11
leukoplakia   108, 108p
   oral hairy   112
lichen planus   109, 110p
lignocaine
   adverse effects
      local   158
      systemic   47
   clinical pharmacology   49
      properties and maximum doses   50t
   precautions   49
   pregnancy and breastfeeding
      risk categorisation   199t
   therapeutic use
      aphthous ulcers   115
      local anaesthesia   158
life support flow chart   187f
lincomycin
   adverse effects   25
   clinical pharmacology   25
   pregnancy and breastfeeding
      risk categorisation   199t
   therapeutic use
      dentoalveolar procedures
         prophylaxis for   141
      endocarditis prophylaxis   138
      odontogenic infections   131
lincosamides
   (see also individual drugs)
   adverse effects   25
   clinical pharmacology   25
   examples of   16t
local anaesthesia   157–9
   complications   158
      local   159
      systemic   47
   definitions   45
   types of   157
local anaesthetics   45–53
   (see also individual drugs)
   adverse effects
      local   158
      systemic   47
         allergy   180
   choice of   48
   clinical pharmacology   45
      properties of groups   46t

local anaesthetics (cont.)
   drugs (individual)   49–52
   vasoconstrictors with   49
local analgesia   *see* local anaesthesia
local analgesics *see* local anaesthetics
   (see also individual drugs)
Ludwig's angina   132

M

macrolides
   (see also individual drugs)
   adverse effects   25
   clinical pharmacology   25
   examples of   16t
   interactions   26
management, principles of   1b, 4
medical emergencies   165–87
   see emergencies (medical)
medical illnesses and dental
   treatment   61–90
   cardiovascular conditions   61
   chronic musculoskeletal disorders   86
   endocrine conditions   70
   head and neck cancer   84
   neurological conditions   79
   psychological and psychiatric
      disorders   88
   respiratory conditions   67
   viral diseases   83
medications
   dental management of patients
      taking   61
mepivacaine
   adverse effects
      local   158
      systemic   47
   clinical pharmacology   52
      properties and maximum doses   51t
   pregnancy and breastfeeding
      risk categorisation   200t
   therapeutic use
      local anaesthesia   158
methaemoglobinaemia
   articaine and   52
   prilocaine and   46, 52
methylprednisolone aceponate
   adverse effects   42
   clinical pharmacology
      potency   40t
   pregnancy and breastfeeding
      risk categorisation   200t
   principles of use   38
   therapeutic use   40t

metronidazole
- adverse effects — 24
- clinical pharmacology — 24
- interactions — 24
- pregnancy and breastfeeding
  - risk categorisation — 200t
- therapeutic use
  - acute ulcerative gingivitis — 100
  - dentoalveolar surgery
    - infection following — 133
  - odontogenic infections — 130, 131

miconazole
- adverse effects — 28
- clinical pharmacology — 27
- interactions — 28
- pregnancy and breastfeeding
  - risk categorisation — 200t
- therapeutic use
  - angular cheilitis — 120
  - candidosis — 119

mometasone furoate
- adverse effects — 42
- clinical pharmacology
  - potency — 40t
- pregnancy and breastfeeding
  - risk categorisation — 200t
- principles of use — 38
- therapeutic use — 40t

morphine
- adverse effects — 34, 35t
- clinical pharmacology — 36
- interactions — 36
- precautions — 36
- pregnancy and breastfeeding
  - risk categorisation — 200t

mouthwashes — 57–60
- (see also individual agents)
- use of alcohol in — 58

mucosal disease — 107–24
- angular cheilitis — 120
- candidosis — 118
- discolourations — 108
- erythema multiforme — 118
- fungal infections — 118
- geographic tongue — 111
- hairy tongue — 111
- lichen planus — 109
- mucositis — 121
- mucous membrane pemphigoid — 117
- oral hairy leukoplakia — 112
- pemphigus vulgaris — 117
- ulcers — 113

mucositis — 121

mucous membrane pemphigoid — 117, 117p

musculoskeletal disorders
- dental issues in patients with — 86

myocardial infarction
- dental issues in patients with — 65
- emergency management — 168, 169b

N

naproxen
- adverse effects — 30, 31t
  - risk factors for gastrointestinal — 32t
- clinical pharmacology — 32
- interactions — 30
- precautions — 30
- pregnancy and breastfeeding
  - risk categorisation — 200t
- principles of use — 29

narcotics — see opioids

needlestick injuries — 83

nerve injuries from local anaesthesia — 159

neurological conditions — 79
- epilepsy — 80
- stroke — 80
- trigeminal neuralgia — 81

neurological emergencies — 176
- seizures — 176
- stroke — 176

neuropathic pain — 145

nitroimidazoles
- (see also individual drugs)
- adverse effects — 24
- clinical pharmacology — 24
- examples of — 16t
- interactions — 24

nonsteroidal anti-inflammatory drugs
- (see also individual drugs)
- adverse effects — 30, 31t
  - risk factors for gastrointestinal — 32t
- interactions — 30
- precautions — 30
- principles of use — 29

NSAIDs — see nonsteroidal anti-inflammatory drugs

nystatin
- adverse effects — 28
- clinical pharmacology — 28
- pregnancy and breastfeeding
  - risk categorisation — 200t
- therapeutic use
  - angular cheilitis — 120
  - candidosis — 120

O

obstruction of the airway 174
  management 174b
  signs of 174
obstructive sleep apnoea
  dental issues in patients with 69
odontogenic infections 127–34
  (see also prophylaxis (antibiotic))
  localised 127
  locations (schematic diagram) 128f
  Ludwig's angina 132
  post–dentoalveolar surgery 132
  spreading 129
    deep 130
    superficial 129
opioids
  adverse effects 34, 35t
  interactions 36
  precautions 36
  principles of use 34
oral hairy leukoplakia 112, 112p
oral lichen planus 109, 110p
oral malodour see halitosis
Oral mucosal disease 107–24
Oral sedation 161–4
osteonecrosis of the jaws 76
  history-taking in relation to 76b
  risk of 77t
osteoporosis 75
  dental issues in patients with 76
osteoradionecrosis 85

P

pain 145
  acute 146
  chronic 146
  management (post-traumatic) 145
    (see also pain management)
    adults 149
    children 151
  types of 145
pain management (post-traumatic) 145–55
  adults 149
  children 151
  strategies 149
  third molar model 154b
palifermin
  pregnancy and breastfeeding
    risk categorisation 200t
  therapeutic use
    mucositis 122
paracetamol
  adverse effects 34
    overdose 34
  clinical pharmacology 33
    third molar model 154b
  interactions 34
  precautions 33
  pregnancy and breastfeeding
    risk categorisation 200t
  principles of use 146
  therapeutic use
    pain, post-treatment
      adults 150
      children 151
paracetamol+codeine
  therapeutic use
    pain, post-treatment (adults) 150
paraesthesia from local anaesthesia 159
pemphigus vulgaris 117
penicillin hypersensitivity 17
penicillin V see phenoxymethylpenicillin
penicillins
  (see also individual drugs and beta lactams)
  adverse effects 21, 22
    hypersensitivity 17
  clinical pharmacology 21, 22
  examples of 16t
  interactions 21
  precautions 21
periodontal abscess 100
periodontal disease 97–101
  hepatitis C and 83
  pathophysiology 97
  xerostomia and 122
periodontitis 98
phenoxymethylpenicillin
  adverse effects 21, 22
  clinical pharmacology 21, 22
  interactions 21
  precautions 21
  pregnancy and breastfeeding
    risk categorisation 200t
  therapeutic use
    dentoalveolar surgery
      infection following 133
      prophylaxis for 141
    odontogenic infections 129, 130
    periodontal abscess 100
pilocarpine
  therapeutic use
    xerostomia 124

plaque
as a cause of caries	91
as a cause of periodontal disease	97
definition	91

polyenes *(see also individual drugs)*
adverse effects	28
clinical pharmacology	28
examples of	16t

Post-treatment pain management 145–55

povidone-iodine
(see also mouthwashes)
adverse effects	60
clinical pharmacology	59
precautions	60
pregnancy and breastfeeding	
risk categorisation	200t

prednisolone
adverse effects	45
adrenal suppression	74
clinical pharmacology	44
dosing	
before dental procedures	75
precautions	
with stressful situations	75
pregnancy and breastfeeding	
risk categorisation	200t
therapeutic use	
Addisonian (adrenal) crisis	179
aphthous ulcers	115
lichen planus	111

prednisone see prednisolone

pregnancy
categorisation of drugs	195
categorisation of individual drugs	197t
drugs and	193
radiographs and	193

prescribing and prescription-writing 5–12
components of a prescription	7
legislation	11
overprescribing	7
principles of	1, 5, 7
underprescribing	7

prescriptions
components of	7
essential information	8
example of	9f
information given to patient	10

prilocaine
adverse effects	
local	158
systemic	47, 52

prilocaine (cont.)
clinical pharmacology	45, 49
properties and maximum doses	50t
precautions	
methaemoglobinaemia	46, 49
pregnancy and breastfeeding	
risk categorisation	200t
therapeutic use	
local anaesthesia	158

principles
of antibiotic use	14b
of diagnosis	1–4
of examination	2
of history-taking	2
of investigations	2
of management	4
of prescribing	1, 5–12
of treatment	1b

procedures (dental)
antibiotic prophylaxis for	140
bacteraemia and	137t
patients taking medications and	
aspirin	63
bisphosphonates	78
warfarin	63
procedure for	64b
relationship between dental procedure and bacteraemia	139f

promethazine
adverse effects	56
clinical pharmacology	56
contraindications	56
precautions	57
pregnancy and breastfeeding	
risk categorisation	200t
therapeutic use	
anaphylactic and anaphylactoid reactions	185b
sedation (children)	153

prophylaxis, antibiotic 135
dental procedures with risk	137t
endocarditis	135
cardiac conditions with risk	136t
prosthetic joint	140
surgery	
dentoalveolar procedures	140
patients with hepatitis C	83

prosthetic joint
prevention of infection	140
dental treatment and	142b

pseudocholinesterase deficiency 46
pseudomembranous candidosis 118
pseudomembranous colitis
antibiotics and	17

psychogenic pain	146
psychological and psychiatric disorders	
dental issues in patients with	88
pulse oximetry	
sedation and	164

R

radiographs and pregnancy	193
radiotherapy of head and neck region	
adverse effects	
mucositis	121
osteoradionecrosis	85
xerostomia	123
dental issues in patients having	85
ranitidine	
therapeutic use	
anaphylactic and anaphylactoid reactions	185b
recurrent aphthous stomatitis	114
regional block anaesthesia	157
Regulations (legislation) relating to drugs and prescriptions	11
resistance to antibiotics	15
respiratory conditions	67
asthma	67
chronic obstructive pulmonary disease	69
obstructive sleep apnoea	69
respiratory emergencies	170
asthma	171
hyperventilation syndrome	170
inhaled objects	172
Reye's syndrome	31
rheumatic fever, prevention of	140
risk–benefit of prescribing	7
roxithromycin	
adverse effects	25
clinical pharmacology	25
interactions	26
pregnancy and breastfeeding risk categorisation	200t

S

salbutamol	
therapeutic use	
anaphylactic and anaphylactoid reactions	185b
asthma	173b
salivary gland agenesis	
xerostomia and	123
salivary gland hypofunction	
	see xerostomia

SCC	*see* squamous cell carcinoma
sedation (oral)	161–4
advantages and disadvantages	161t
assessment for	161
drugs used for	162
instructions for patients	163b
management of	163
preparation for	162
sedatives	53
seizures	176
management	177b
Sjögren's syndrome	
xerostomia and	123
somatoform pain	146
sporting authorities and drugs	191
squamous cell carcinoma	109p
stent placement	
dental issues in patients with	66
stomatitis (viral)	115
stroke	176
dental issues in patients with	80
emergency management	176b
surgery	*see* procedures (dental)
swallowed objects	173
management	174b
prevention	172
syncope	166
management	167b

T

teicoplanin	
adverse effects	25
clinical pharmacology	24
pregnancy and breastfeeding risk categorisation	200t
therapeutic use	
endocarditis prophylaxis	139
temazepam	
adverse effects	54
clinical pharmacology	55
contraindications	54
precautions	54
pregnancy and breastfeeding risk categorisation	200t
therapeutic use	
sedation	162
temporomandibular disorders	
dental issues in patients with	87
terbutaline	
therapeutic use	
anaphylactic and anaphylactoid reactions	185b

tetracyclines
(see also individual drugs)
adverse effects — 26
children and — 26
clinical pharmacology — 26
examples of — 16t
interactions — 27
precautions — 26
pregnancy and breastfeeding — 26
risk categorisation — 201t
third molar model for pain management — 154b
thymidine analogues
(see also individual drugs)
clinical pharmacology — 29
examples of — 17t
thyroid disorders — 72
hyperthyroidism — 73
hypothyroidism — 72
thyrotoxicosis
dental issues in patients with — 73
tinidazole
adverse effects — 24
clinical pharmacology — 24
interactions — 24
pregnancy and breastfeeding
risk categorisation — 201t
tolerance (drug) — 57
tooth decay
modifying factors — 92
pathophysiology — 91
stages (schematic diagram) — 128f
treatment — 92
xerostomia and — 122
tooth discolouration with tetracyclines — 26
tooth extraction
infection following — 141
tooth infections
see odontogenic infections
tranexamic acid
administration
tranexamic mouthwash protocol 64b
pregnancy and breastfeeding
risk categorisation — 201t
therapeutic use
surgery in patients taking warfarin — 64b
transient ischemic attack — 176
management — 176b
treatment, principles of — 1b
trench mouth — 99
with HIV — 100

triamcinolone acetonide
adverse effects — 42
clinical pharmacology
potency — 40t
pregnancy and breastfeeding
risk categorisation — 201t
principles of use — 38
therapeutic use — 40t
aphthous ulcers — 115
lichen planus — 110
triclosan *(see also mouthwashes)*
clinical pharmacology — 60
pregnancy and breastfeeding
risk categorisation — 201t
therapeutic use
halitosis (oral malodour) — 105
tricyclic antidepressants
adverse effects
xerostomia — 122
trigeminal nerve injury — 82
trigeminal neuralgia
dental issues in patients with — 81
trimeprazine
adverse effects — 56
clinical pharmacology — 56
contraindications — 56
precautions — 56
pregnancy and breastfeeding
risk categorisation — 201t
trismus — 130
local anaesthesia and — 159

U
ulcers (mouth) — 113–18, 113p
aphthous — 114
causes of — 114t
viral — 115
urticaria — 181
management — 182b

V
valaciclovir
clinical pharmacology — 28
pregnancy and breastfeeding
risk categorisation — 201t
vancomycin
adverse effects — 25
clinical pharmacology — 24
pregnancy and breastfeeding
risk categorisation — 201t
therapeutic use
endocarditis prophylaxis — 138

vasoconstrictors	52–3
(see also individual drugs)	
use of with local anaesthetics	49
vasovagal syncope	166
management	167b
Vincent's disease	99
with HIV	100
viral diseases	
hepatitis	83
human immunodeficiency virus	84
ulcers	115
viral hepatitis	
dental issues in patients with	83
viral ulcers	115
voriconazole	
adverse effects	28
clinical pharmacology	27
interactions	28
pregnancy and breastfeeding	
risk categorisation	201t

W

warfarin	
dental management of patients taking	62, 63
procedure for patients requiring oral surgery	64b

X

xerostomia	122
as cause of mucositis	121
caries and	122
periodontal disease and	122

Z

zinc	
pregnancy and breastfeeding risk categorisation	201t
therapeutic use	
halitosis	105

Request for comment on guidelines

Help us to help you

As the final user of this volume, you can give us valuable advice about the content, layout and usability of this book. Your comments will be most appreciated and will be considered during the preparation of the next edition.

Therapeutic Guidelines: Oral and Dental version 1, 2007

Comments _____
_____
_____
_____
_____
_____
_____
_____
_____
_____

Name _____

Address _____
_____

Detach this page and return to:

Therapeutic Guidelines Limited
Ground floor, 23–47 Villiers Street
North Melbourne, Victoria 3051
Australia

Freecall: 1800 061 260
Email: evaluation@tg.com.au